SUPER EASY LOW-CARB DIABETIC COOKBOOK FOR BEGINNERS

Ultimate Guide To 2000 Days Of Delicious Low-Carb, Low-Sugar Diabetic-Friendly Recipes For Pre-Diabetes, Type 2 Diabetes And Newly Diagnosed With A 31-Day Meal Plan

Marcus Baron

Table of Contents

COPYRIGHT © 2023

CHAPTER ONE

Understanding Low-Carb Diabetic Cooking

Introduction to Low-Carb Diabetic Diet

A low-carb diabetic diet is a nutritional approach that focuses on minimizing carbohydrate intake to manage blood sugar levels effectively. For individuals with diabetes, particularly type 2 diabetes, controlling carbohydrate consumption can be crucial in regulating blood glucose levels, reducing the need for medication, and improving overall health outcomes. This section will delve into the rationale behind adopting a low-carb approach for diabetes management, the fundamentals of carbohydrate counting, and the impact of low-carb eating on blood sugar control.

Benefits of a Low-Carb Approach for Diabetes

The benefits of adopting a low-carb diet for individuals with diabetes are multifaceted and well-documented. One of the primary advantages is its ability to help regulate blood sugar levels more effectively compared to higher-carb diets. By limiting the intake of carbohydrates, which are broken down into glucose during digestion, individuals can prevent sharp spikes in blood sugar levels, thus reducing the need for insulin or other glucose-lowering medications.

Moreover, low-carb diets have been associated with improvements in insulin sensitivity, which is particularly beneficial for individuals with insulin resistance, a hallmark of type 2 diabetes. By reducing the demand for insulin, cells become more responsive to its effects, facilitating better blood sugar control and potentially reducing the risk of complications associated with diabetes, such as cardiovascular disease and neuropathy.

Additionally, low-carb diets often lead to weight loss or weight maintenance, which can be advantageous for individuals with diabetes, as excess body weight is a significant risk factor for insulin resistance and complications related to diabetes. By promoting satiety and reducing overall calorie intake, low-carb diets can help individuals achieve and maintain a healthy weight, further improving glycemic control and metabolic health.

Furthermore, low-carb diets have been shown to have favorable effects on various cardiovascular risk factors, such as blood pressure, triglycerides, and HDL cholesterol levels. By promoting a favorable lipid profile and reducing inflammation, low-carb eating may lower the risk of heart disease, a common comorbidity in individuals with diabetes.

Basics of Carbohydrate Counting

Carbohydrate counting is a fundamental aspect of managing diabetes, especially for those who choose to follow a low-carb diet. It involves estimating the amount of carbohydrates in foods and beverages and adjusting insulin doses or meal plans accordingly to maintain stable blood sugar levels.

To effectively count carbohydrates, individuals need to understand which foods contain carbohydrates and how different types of carbohydrates affect blood sugar levels. Carbohydrates are primarily found in foods such as grains, starchy vegetables, fruits, dairy products, and sweets. However, not all carbohydrates are created equal.

Fiber, for example, is a type of carbohydrate that is not fully digested and absorbed by the body, leading to a slower and more gradual increase in blood sugar levels. Therefore, foods high in fiber, such as non-starchy vegetables and whole grains, have a lower impact on blood sugar compared to refined carbohydrates like white bread or sugary snacks.

Furthermore, individuals with diabetes need to be mindful of the glycemic index (GI) of foods, which measures how quickly a particular food raises blood sugar levels. Foods with a high GI, such as white rice or sugary cereals, cause rapid spikes in blood sugar, while those with a low GI, such as legumes or nuts, result in more gradual increases.

By incorporating low-GI foods into their meals, individuals can help minimize post-meal blood sugar spikes and achieve better glycemic control. Carbohydrate counting empowers individuals with diabetes to make informed choices about their food intake, allowing them to manage their condition effectively and optimize their overall health outcomes.

How Low-Carb Eating Affects Blood Sugar

The impact of low-carb eating on blood sugar levels is a central aspect of diabetes management. By reducing carbohydrate intake, individuals can minimize the amount of glucose entering their bloodstream, leading to more stable and predictable blood sugar levels throughout the day.

When carbohydrates are consumed, they are broken down into glucose and absorbed into the bloodstream, causing blood sugar levels to rise. In response, the pancreas releases insulin, a hormone that helps transport glucose from the bloodstream into cells, where it can be used for energy or stored for later use.

However, in individuals with diabetes, this process is impaired, either due to insufficient insulin production (type 1 diabetes) or ineffective use of insulin by the body (type 2 diabetes). As a result, blood sugar levels remain elevated, leading to hyperglycemia, which can have detrimental effects on health if left uncontrolled.

By limiting carbohydrate intake, individuals can reduce the demand for insulin and alleviate the burden on their pancreas. This can be particularly beneficial for individuals with type 2 diabetes, as it may improve insulin sensitivity and reduce the risk of complications associated with chronic hyperglycemia.

Moreover, low-carb eating can help prevent the sharp spikes and crashes in blood sugar levels commonly experienced after consuming high-carb meals. By choosing foods that have a minimal impact on blood sugar, individuals can maintain more stable energy levels throughout the day and avoid the fatigue and hunger pangs associated with fluctuating blood sugar levels.

Additionally, low-carb diets have been shown to promote ketosis, a metabolic state in which the body burns fat for fuel in the absence of sufficient carbohydrates. Ketones, byproducts of fat metabolism, can serve as an alternative energy source for cells, including the brain, reducing the body's reliance on glucose for fuel. This can be particularly advantageous for individuals with diabetes, as it may help improve insulin sensitivity and promote weight loss.

In summary, low-carb eating can have significant benefits for individuals with diabetes, including better blood sugar control, improved insulin sensitivity, and reduced risk of complications. By understanding the principles of carbohydrate counting and the effects of low-carb eating on blood sugar levels, individuals can take control of their diabetes and improve their overall health outcomes.

Essential Ingredients for Low-Carb Cooking

Low-Carb Vegetables: A Foundation for Meals

Low-carb vegetables are an essential component of a low-carb diet, providing essential nutrients, fiber, and flavor without significantly impacting blood sugar levels. Incorporating a variety of non-starchy vegetables into meals can add volume, texture, and color while keeping carbohydrate intake in check.

Non-starchy vegetables are rich in vitamins, minerals, and antioxidants, making them valuable additions to any diet, especially for individuals with diabetes who may have increased nutrient needs or deficiencies. Some examples of low-carb vegetables include leafy greens (spinach, kale, lettuce), cruciferous vegetables (broccoli, cauliflower, Brussels sprouts), and other colorful options like bell peppers, zucchini, and eggplant.

Lean Proteins: Building Blocks of Low-Carb Dishes

Protein is a crucial macronutrient for overall health and satiety, making it an essential component of low-carb meals. Lean protein sources, such as poultry, fish, tofu, and legumes, provide amino acids, the building blocks of protein, without adding significant amounts of carbohydrates or saturated fat.

Incorporating lean proteins into meals can help promote feelings of fullness and satisfaction, making it easier to adhere to a low-carb diet and control calorie intake. Additionally, protein plays a key role in muscle maintenance and repair, particularly important for individuals with diabetes who may be at risk of muscle loss or weakness.

Healthy Fats: Flavor Enhancers and Satiety Boosters

Healthy fats are an integral part of a low-carb diet, providing flavor, texture, and satiety without significantly affecting blood sugar levels. Incorporating sources of healthy fats, such as avocado, nuts, seeds, olive oil, and fatty fish, into meals can enhance taste and satisfaction while promoting heart health and weight management.

Unlike carbohydrates, which can cause rapid fluctuations in blood sugar levels, fats are digested and absorbed slowly, resulting in a gradual and sustained release of energy. This can help prevent blood sugar spikes and crashes, providing a more stable source of fuel for the body.

Moreover, fats are essential for the absorption of fat-soluble vitamins (A, D, E, K) and play a critical role in hormone production, cell membrane structure, and brain function. By including a variety of healthy fats in their diet, individuals can support overall health and well-being while enjoying delicious and satisfying meals.

Tools and Equipment for Low-Carb Kitchen

Essential Kitchen Gadgets for Easy Cooking

Equipping your kitchen with the right tools and gadgets can make low-carb cooking more convenient, efficient, and enjoyable. From food processors and spiralizers to air fryers and immersion blenders, there are numerous gadgets available to help streamline meal preparation and enhance culinary creativity.

Food processors are versatile appliances that can chop, puree, and blend ingredients, making them ideal for preparing sauces, dips, and homemade nut butters. Spiralizers are handy tools for turning vegetables like zucchini and sweet potatoes into noodles or ribbons, offering a low-carb alternative to traditional pasta.

Air fryers use hot air circulation to cook food quickly and evenly, producing crispy and delicious results with minimal oil. Immersion blenders are compact and easy to use, perfect for blending soups, sauces, and smoothies directly in the pot or container.

Stocking a Low-Carb Pantry

Maintaining a well-stocked pantry is essential for low-carb cooking, ensuring you have the necessary ingredients on hand to prepare delicious and nutritious meals. When stocking your pantry, focus on low-carb staples such as nuts, seeds, nut flours, coconut flour, almond meal, and low-carb sweeteners like stevia or erythritol.

Additionally, keep a variety of herbs, spices, and condiments on hand to add flavor to your dishes without relying on high-carb sauces or seasonings. Ingredients like garlic, ginger, cumin, paprika, and vinegar can enhance the taste of your meals while providing health benefits.

Don't forget to include pantry essentials like canned tuna, salmon, and chicken, as well as shelf-stable options like broth, canned tomatoes, and coconut milk. These items can serve as the foundation for quick and easy meals, especially when fresh ingredients are not readily available.

Meal Prep Tips for Quick Low-Carb Meals

Meal prep is a key strategy for staying on track with a low-carb diet, allowing you to prepare healthy meals in advance and avoid the temptation of convenience foods or takeout. When meal prepping for a low-carb diet, focus on batch-cooking proteins, vegetables, and grains (if desired) to have on hand throughout the week.

Start by planning your meals and snacks for the week ahead, taking into account your schedule, dietary preferences, and nutritional goals. Choose recipes that are easy to prepare in large batches and can be stored and reheated easily, such as soups, stews, casseroles, and stir-fries.

Once you have your meal plan in place, dedicate some time each week to grocery shopping and meal prep. Wash, chop, and portion out vegetables, cook proteins, and assemble meals in individual containers for grab-and-go convenience.

Consider investing in reusable containers and meal prep accessories like portion-control containers, silicone muffin cups, and compartmentalized lunch boxes to make meal prep even more efficient and organized. By setting aside a few hours each week to prepare and portion out your meals, you can save time, money, and stress while sticking to your low-carb diet goals.

In conclusion, understanding low-carb diabetic cooking involves grasping the benefits of a low-carb approach for diabetes management, mastering the basics of carbohydrate counting, and recognizing how low-carb eating affects blood sugar levels. Essential ingredients for low-carb cooking include low-carb vegetables, lean proteins, and healthy fats, while essential tools and equipment for the low-carb kitchen include kitchen gadgets, a well-stocked pantry, and meal prep tips for quick low-carb meals. By incorporating these principles into your cooking routine, you can enjoy delicious, nutritious, and blood sugar-friendly meals that support your health and well-being.

CHAPTER TWO

Quick and Easy Low-Carb Breakfasts

When it comes to starting the day on the right foot, a nutritious breakfast is key, especially for those following a low-carb diet. In this section, we'll explore a variety of quick and easy low-carb breakfast options that are not only delicious but also satisfying and energizing.

High-Protein Breakfasts to Start the Day Right

High-protein breakfasts are an excellent choice for those looking to fuel their morning and stay satisfied until their next meal. Protein helps to stabilize blood sugar levels and promotes feelings of fullness, making it an essential component of a low-carb breakfast.

Scrambled Eggs with Spinach and Feta

Scrambled eggs with spinach and feta cheese is a simple yet flavorful breakfast option that can be prepared in minutes. To make this dish, start by whisking eggs in a bowl and seasoning with salt and pepper. In a non-stick skillet, sauté fresh spinach until wilted, then add the beaten eggs and cook until scrambled. Crumble feta cheese over the eggs and serve hot, garnished with fresh herbs if desired. This dish is rich in protein, vitamins, and minerals, making it an excellent choice for a low-carb breakfast.

Greek Yogurt Parfait with Berries and Almonds

Greek yogurt parfait with berries and almonds is a refreshing and satisfying breakfast option that's packed with protein and fiber. To make this parfait, layer Greek yogurt with fresh berries (such as strawberries, blueberries, or raspberries) and sliced almonds in a glass or bowl. Repeat the layers until you reach the top, then drizzle with a small amount of honey or a sprinkle of cinnamon for added sweetness. This breakfast is not only delicious but also provides a good balance of nutrients to kick-start your day.

Veggie Omelet with Avocado Slices

A veggie omelet with avocado slices is a nutrient-dense and filling breakfast option that's perfect for those following a low-carb diet. To make this omelet, sauté your favorite vegetables (such as bell peppers, onions, mushrooms, and tomatoes) in a non-stick skillet until tender. Pour beaten eggs over the vegetables and cook until set, then fold the omelet in half and serve with sliced avocado on top. This breakfast is rich in protein, healthy fats, and fiber, making it a satisfying and nutritious way to start your day.

Low-Carb Breakfast Bakes and Casseroles

Low-carb breakfast bakes and casseroles are convenient options for meal prep or feeding a crowd. These dishes can be prepared in advance and reheated throughout the week, making them ideal for busy mornings or lazy weekends.

Crustless Quiche with Bacon and Cheddar

A crustless quiche with bacon and cheddar cheese is a hearty and flavorful breakfast option that's perfect for brunch or meal prep. To make this quiche, start by cooking bacon until crisp, then crumble it into a greased baking dish. In a bowl, whisk together eggs, cream, shredded cheddar cheese, and your favorite seasonings. Pour the egg mixture over the bacon in the baking dish and bake until set and golden brown. This crustless quiche is low in carbs and high in protein, making it a satisfying and delicious breakfast choice.

Baked Egg Muffins with Ham and Cheese

Baked egg muffins with ham and cheese are portable and customizable breakfast options that can be enjoyed on the go. To make these muffins, whisk together eggs, diced ham, shredded cheese, and chopped vegetables (such as bell peppers, onions, and spinach) in a bowl. Divide the mixture evenly among greased muffin cups and bake until set and golden brown. These egg muffins are packed with protein and can be stored in the refrigerator or freezer for quick and easy breakfasts throughout the week.

Spinach and Mushroom Breakfast Casserole

A spinach and mushroom breakfast casserole is a nutritious and satisfying dish that's perfect for feeding a crowd. To make this casserole, sauté fresh spinach and sliced mushrooms in a skillet until tender, then transfer to a greased baking dish. In a bowl, whisk together eggs, milk, shredded cheese, and seasonings, then pour the mixture over the spinach and mushrooms in the baking dish. Bake until set and golden brown, then slice and serve. This breakfast casserole is low in carbs and high in protein and fiber, making it a filling and delicious option for any morning.

Energizing Smoothies and Shakes

Energizing smoothies and shakes are quick and convenient breakfast options that can be customized to suit your taste preferences and nutritional needs. Packed with protein, vitamins, and minerals, these beverages are perfect for busy mornings or post-workout refueling.

Green Keto Smoothie with Avocado and Spinach

A green keto smoothie with avocado and spinach is a refreshing and nutrient-dense breakfast option that's perfect for those following a low-carb diet. To make this smoothie, blend together avocado, spinach, coconut milk, protein powder, and a handful of ice until smooth and creamy. You can also add a splash of lemon juice or a few drops of stevia for extra flavor. This smoothie is rich in healthy fats, fiber, and protein, making it a satisfying and energizing way to start your day.

Berry Protein Shake with Unsweetened Almond Milk

A berry protein shake with unsweetened almond milk is a delicious and nutritious breakfast option that's perfect for busy mornings. To make this shake, blend together mixed berries (such as strawberries, blueberries, and raspberries), unsweetened almond milk, protein powder, and a handful of ice until smooth and creamy. You can also add a tablespoon of chia seeds or flaxseeds for added fiber and omega-3 fatty acids. This protein shake is low in carbs and high in protein, making it a great choice for anyone looking to fuel their day.

Coffee Protein Smoothie with MCT Oil

A coffee protein smoothie with MCT oil is a delicious and invigorating breakfast option that's perfect for coffee lovers. To make this smoothie, blend together cold brew coffee, protein powder, MCT oil, unsweetened almond milk, and a handful of ice until smooth and frothy. You can also add a dash of cinnamon or cocoa powder for extra flavor. This smoothie is rich in caffeine, protein, and healthy fats, making it a great way to kick-start your day and keep you energized until lunchtime.

In conclusion, these quick and easy low-carb breakfast options are perfect for busy mornings or leisurely weekends when you want to start your day off right. Whether you prefer high-protein dishes like scrambled eggs or Greek yogurt parfaits, savory breakfast bakes and casseroles, or energizing smoothies and shakes, there's something for everyone to enjoy while staying on track with your low-carb goals.

CHAPTER THREE

Simple Low-Carb Lunch Ideas

Finding simple and satisfying low-carb lunch options can be easy with the right recipes and ingredients. In this section, we'll explore a variety of lunch ideas that are delicious, nutritious, and perfect for keeping you fueled throughout the day.

Fresh and Flavorful Salad Bowls

Salad bowls are versatile, customizable, and perfect for incorporating a variety of fresh ingredients into your lunch. Whether you prefer classic combinations or unique flavor profiles, there's a salad bowl option to suit every taste preference.

Grilled Chicken Caesar Salad with Parmesan Crisps

A grilled chicken Caesar salad with Parmesan crisps is a satisfying and flavorful lunch option that's perfect for anyone following a low-carb diet. Start by grilling chicken breasts seasoned with salt, pepper, and your favorite herbs or spices. Meanwhile, prepare a bed of crisp romaine lettuce and toss with Caesar dressing until well coated. Top the salad with grilled chicken slices, shaved Parmesan cheese, and homemade Parmesan crisps for added crunch. This salad is packed with protein, fiber, and healthy fats, making it a nutritious and delicious option for lunch.

Cobb Salad with Avocado and Blue Cheese

A Cobb salad with avocado and blue cheese is a hearty and satisfying lunch option that's perfect for those following a low-carb diet. To make this salad, start by arranging a bed of mixed greens in a large bowl. Top with diced grilled chicken, crispy bacon, hard-boiled eggs, cherry tomatoes, avocado slices, and crumbled blue cheese. Drizzle with your favorite vinaigrette or dressing, then toss until well combined. This salad is rich in protein, healthy fats, and vitamins, making it a nutritious and filling option for lunch.

Mediterranean Salad with Olives and Feta

A Mediterranean salad with olives and feta cheese is a refreshing and flavorful lunch option that's perfect for anyone following a low-carb diet. To make this salad, start by combining mixed greens, cherry tomatoes, cucumber slices, red onion slices, Kalamata olives, and crumbled feta cheese in a large bowl. Drizzle with olive oil and balsamic vinegar, then season with salt, pepper, and dried oregano to taste. Toss until well combined, then serve immediately. This salad is packed with antioxidants, vitamins, and minerals, making it a nutritious and delicious option for lunch.

Low-Carb Wraps and Sandwiches

Low-carb wraps and sandwiches are convenient options for lunch on the go or enjoying at home. By swapping out traditional bread for low-carb alternatives like lettuce leaves or collard greens, you can enjoy all your favorite fillings without the extra carbs.

Turkey Lettuce Wraps with Hummus

Turkey lettuce wraps with hummus are a quick and easy lunch option that's perfect for anyone following a low-carb diet. To make these wraps, start by spreading a generous dollop of hummus onto large lettuce leaves (such as butter lettuce or iceberg lettuce). Top with sliced turkey breast, sliced cucumber, shredded carrots, and sprouts or microgreens. Roll up the lettuce leaves tightly, then secure with toothpicks if needed. These wraps are packed with protein, fiber, and flavor, making them a nutritious and satisfying option for lunch.

Tuna Salad Collard Green Wraps

Tuna salad collard green wraps are a light and refreshing lunch option that's perfect for anyone following a low-carb diet. To make these wraps, start by preparing a simple tuna salad with canned tuna, mayonnaise, diced celery, red onion, and Dijon mustard. Spread the tuna salad onto large collard green leaves, then add sliced avocado, shredded carrot, and cucumber slices. Roll up the collard green leaves tightly, then slice in half if desired. These wraps are rich in protein, healthy fats, and vitamins, making them a nutritious and satisfying option for lunch.

Caprese Sandwich with Tomato, Mozzarella, and Basil

A Caprese sandwich with tomato, mozzarella, and basil is a classic and delicious lunch option that's perfect for anyone following a low-carb diet. To make this sandwich, start by layering thinly sliced tomato, fresh mozzarella cheese, and basil leaves on a large lettuce leaf or low-carb wrap. Drizzle with balsamic glaze or olive oil, then season with salt and pepper to taste. Fold the lettuce leaf or wrap over the filling to form a sandwich, then serve immediately. This sandwich is packed with flavor and nutrients, making it a nutritious and satisfying option for lunch.

Hearty Soups and Stews

Soups and stews are comforting and nourishing lunch options that can be prepared in advance and enjoyed throughout the week. By choosing low-carb ingredients like vegetables, protein, and broth, you can create delicious and satisfying meals that won't derail your low-carb goals.

Keto Chicken and Vegetable Soup

Keto chicken and vegetable soup is a hearty and comforting lunch option that's perfect for anyone following a low-carb diet. To make this soup, start by sautéing diced onions, carrots, celery, and garlic in a large pot until softened. Add diced chicken breast, chicken broth, diced tomatoes, and your favorite herbs and spices (such as thyme, rosemary, and bay leaves). Simmer the soup until the chicken is cooked through and the vegetables are tender. Serve hot, garnished with fresh parsley or grated Parmesan cheese. This soup is rich in protein, fiber, and vitamins, making it a nutritious and filling option for lunch.

Beef and Broccoli Stir-Fry Soup

Beef and broccoli stir-fry soup is a flavorful and satisfying lunch option that's perfect for anyone following a low-carb diet. To make this soup, start by marinating thinly sliced beef in a mixture of soy sauce, garlic, ginger, and sesame oil. Sauté the marinated beef in a large pot until browned, then add chopped broccoli florets, beef broth, and additional soy sauce to taste. Simmer the soup until the beef is cooked through and the broccoli is tender. Serve hot, garnished with sliced green onions or sesame seeds. This soup is packed with protein, fiber, and flavor, making it a nutritious and delicious option for lunch.

Cauliflower and Bacon Chowder

Cauliflower and bacon chowder is a creamy and comforting lunch option that's perfect for anyone following a low-carb diet. To make this chowder, start by cooking diced bacon in a large pot until crispy. Remove the bacon from the pot and set aside, leaving the rendered fat in the pot. Add chopped cauliflower, diced onions, celery, and garlic to the pot, and sauté until softened. Add chicken broth and simmer until the cauliflower is tender. Use an immersion blender to puree the soup until smooth, then stir in heavy cream and cooked bacon pieces. Season with salt, pepper, and chopped fresh herbs to taste. This chowder is rich in flavor and nutrients, making it a satisfying and delicious option for lunch.

In conclusion, these simple low-carb lunch ideas are perfect for anyone looking to enjoy delicious and satisfying meals while staying on track with their dietary goals. Whether you prefer fresh and flavorful salad bowls, low-carb wraps and sandwiches, or hearty soups and stews, there's something for everyone to enjoy while maintaining a low-carb lifestyle.

CHAPTER FOUR

Easy Low-Carb Dinners for Busy Nights

On hectic evenings, preparing a nutritious low-carb dinner doesn't have to be complicated. With these simple yet delicious recipes, you can whip up satisfying meals in no time, perfect for busy nights when you need something quick and easy.

Flavorful Low-Carb Stir-Fries

Stir-fries are a fantastic option for busy nights because they're quick to prepare and infinitely customizable. Packed with protein and vegetables, these dishes are both nutritious and satisfying.

Shrimp Stir-Fry with Broccoli and Bell Peppers

This shrimp stir-fry with broccoli and bell peppers is a light and flavorful dish that comes together in minutes. Start by heating a wok or large skillet over high heat and adding a splash of oil. Add peeled and deveined shrimp to the pan and stir-fry until pink and opaque. Remove the shrimp from the pan and set aside. In the same pan, add chopped broccoli florets and sliced bell peppers, along with minced garlic and ginger. Stir-fry until the vegetables are tender-crisp, then return the shrimp to the pan. Drizzle with soy sauce and sesame oil, then toss everything together until well combined. Serve hot over cauliflower rice for a low-carb twist on a classic stir-fry.

Beef and Vegetable Stir-Fry with Cauliflower Rice

This beef and vegetable stir-fry with cauliflower rice is a hearty and satisfying meal that's perfect for busy nights. Start by thinly slicing flank steak against the grain and marinating it in a mixture of soy sauce, garlic, and ginger. Meanwhile, chop your favorite vegetables, such as bell peppers, snap peas, and carrots. Heat a wok or large skillet over high heat and add the marinated beef, stirring constantly until browned. Remove the beef from the pan and set aside. In the same pan, add the chopped vegetables and stir-fry until tender-crisp. Return the beef to the pan and toss everything together until well combined. Serve hot over cauliflower rice for a low-carb alternative to traditional rice.

Tofu and Mushroom Stir-Fry with Snap Peas

This tofu and mushroom stir-fry with snap peas is a vegetarian-friendly option that's both nutritious and delicious. Start by pressing firm tofu to remove excess moisture, then cut it into cubes. Heat a wok or large skillet over medium-high heat and add a splash of oil. Add sliced mushrooms to the pan and cook until browned and tender. Remove the mushrooms from the pan and set aside. In the same pan, add the cubed tofu and stir-fry until golden brown on all sides. Add snap peas and minced garlic to the pan, along with a drizzle of soy sauce and sesame oil. Stir-fry until the snap peas are bright green and tender-crisp, then return the mushrooms to the pan. Toss everything together until well combined, then serve hot over cauliflower rice or noodles for a satisfying low-carb meal.

Simple Sheet Pan Meals

Sheet pan meals are a lifesaver on busy nights because they require minimal prep and cleanup. With just a few ingredients and a single pan, you can create flavorful and nutritious dinners that the whole family will love.

Lemon Herb Baked Salmon with Asparagus

This lemon herb baked salmon with asparagus is a light and refreshing dish that's perfect for busy nights. Start by preheating your oven to 400°F (200°C) and lining a baking sheet with parchment paper. Place salmon fillets on one side of the baking sheet and arrange trimmed asparagus spears on the other side. Drizzle everything with olive oil and season with salt, pepper, minced garlic, and fresh herbs like dill or parsley. Squeeze fresh lemon juice over the salmon and asparagus, then bake in the preheated oven for 12-15 minutes, or until the salmon is cooked through and the asparagus is tender. Serve hot with additional lemon wedges for squeezing.

Herb-Roasted Chicken Thighs with Brussels Sprouts

These herb-roasted chicken thighs with Brussels sprouts are a comforting and satisfying meal that's perfect for busy nights. Start by preheating your oven to 425°F (220°C) and lining a baking sheet with parchment paper. Arrange bone-in, skin-on chicken thighs on one side of the baking sheet and trim and halve Brussels sprouts on the other side. Drizzle everything with olive oil and season with salt, pepper, and dried herbs like thyme or rosemary. Toss everything together until well coated, then spread out in an even layer on the baking sheet. Bake in the preheated oven for 25-30 minutes, or until the chicken is cooked through and the Brussels sprouts are caramelized and tender. Serve hot with your favorite low-carb side dish.

Sausage and Veggie Sheet Pan Dinner

This sausage and veggie sheet pan dinner is a hearty and flavorful meal that's perfect for busy nights. Start by preheating your oven to 400°F (200°C) and lining a baking sheet with parchment paper. Arrange sliced sausage (such as Italian sausage or chicken sausage) on one side of the baking sheet and chopped vegetables (such as bell peppers, onions, and zucchini) on the other side. Drizzle everything with olive oil and season with salt, pepper, and dried herbs like oregano or basil. Toss everything together until well coated, then spread out in an even layer on the baking sheet. Bake in the preheated oven for 20-25 minutes, or until the sausage is cooked through and the vegetables are tender and caramelized. Serve hot with a side of cauliflower rice or mashed cauliflower for a complete low-carb meal.

Comforting Low-Carb Casseroles

Casseroles are a classic comfort food that can easily be adapted to fit a low-carb lifestyle. With hearty ingredients like meat, vegetables, and cheese, these dishes are satisfying and delicious.

Zucchini Lasagna with Ground Turkey and Ricotta

This zucchini lasagna with ground turkey and ricotta is a lighter take on the classic Italian dish that's perfect for busy nights. Start by preheating your oven to 375°F (190°C) and greasing a 9x13-inch baking dish. Slice zucchini lengthwise into thin strips using a mandoline slicer or sharp knife. Arrange a layer of zucchini slices in the bottom of the prepared baking dish, then top with cooked ground turkey, marinara sauce, and dollops of ricotta cheese. Repeat the layers until all the ingredients are used up, then sprinkle shredded mozzarella cheese over the top. Cover the baking dish with foil and bake in the preheated oven for 30 minutes, then remove the foil and bake for an additional 15 minutes, or until the cheese is bubbly and golden brown. Let cool for a few minutes before slicing and serving.

Cauliflower Mac and Cheese with Bacon

This cauliflower mac and cheese with bacon is a comforting and indulgent dish that's perfect for busy nights. Start by preheating your oven to 375°F (190°C) and greasing a 9x13-inch baking dish. Cook cauliflower florets in boiling water until tender, then drain and set aside. In a large skillet, cook diced bacon until crispy, then remove from the skillet and set aside. In the same skillet, melt butter and whisk in almond flour to form a roux. Gradually whisk in unsweetened almond milk until smooth and creamy, then stir in shredded cheddar cheese until melted and combined. Season with salt, pepper, and garlic powder to taste. Add the cooked cauliflower and crispy bacon to the cheese sauce, then transfer to the prepared baking dish. Sprinkle crushed pork rinds over the top for added crunch, then bake in the preheated oven for 20-25 minutes, or until bubbly and golden brown. Let cool for a few minutes before serving.

Eggplant Parmesan Bake with Mozzarella and Marinara

This eggplant Parmesan bake with mozzarella and marinara is a comforting and satisfying dish that's perfect for busy nights. Start by preheating your oven to 375°F (190°C) and greasing a 9x13-inch baking dish. Slice eggplant into thin rounds and arrange in a single layer on the bottom of the prepared baking dish. Top with marinara sauce, shredded mozzarella cheese, and grated Parmesan cheese. Repeat the layers until all the ingredients are used up, then sprinkle Italian seasoning over the top. Cover the baking dish with foil and bake in the preheated oven for 30 minutes, then remove the foil and bake for an additional 15 minutes, or until the cheese is bubbly and golden brown. Let cool for a few minutes before serving.

In conclusion, these easy low-carb dinners are perfect for busy nights when you need something quick and satisfying. Whether you prefer flavorful stir-fries, simple sheet pan meals, or comforting casseroles, there's something for everyone to enjoy while staying on track with their low-carb goals.

CHAPTER FIVE

Tasty Low-Carb Side Dishes

Low-carb side dishes can complement any meal, adding flavor, texture, and nutrition to your plate. From simple roasted vegetables to flavorful cauliflower creations and fresh salads, there's a wide variety of options to choose from that will satisfy your taste buds and support your low-carb lifestyle.

Simple Roasted Vegetables

Roasting vegetables is a delicious way to bring out their natural flavors and textures while keeping them low in carbs. With just a few simple ingredients and minimal prep time, you can create tasty side dishes that are perfect for any meal.

Garlic Parmesan Roasted Broccoli

Garlic parmesan roasted broccoli is a flavorful and satisfying side dish that's perfect for any low-carb meal. To make this dish, start by preheating your oven to 425°F (220°C) and lining a baking sheet with parchment paper. Toss broccoli florets with olive oil, minced garlic, grated parmesan cheese, salt, and pepper until well coated. Spread the broccoli out in an even layer on the prepared baking sheet and roast in the preheated oven for 20-25 minutes, or until the broccoli is tender and caramelized. Serve hot as a delicious side dish that's sure to impress.

Lemon Herb Roasted Brussels Sprouts

Lemon herb roasted Brussels sprouts are a bright and flavorful side dish that pairs perfectly with any protein. To make this dish, start by preheating your oven to 400°F (200°C) and lining a baking sheet with parchment paper. Trim the ends off Brussels sprouts and cut them in half, then toss them with olive oil, lemon zest, minced garlic, chopped fresh herbs (such as thyme or rosemary), salt, and pepper until well coated. Spread the Brussels sprouts out in an even layer on the prepared baking sheet and roast in the preheated oven for 20-25 minutes, or until golden brown and crispy. Serve hot with a squeeze of lemon juice for extra brightness.

Balsamic Roasted Asparagus with Cherry Tomatoes

Balsamic roasted asparagus with cherry tomatoes is a vibrant and flavorful side dish that's perfect for spring and summer meals. To make this dish, start by preheating your oven to 425°F (220°C) and lining a baking sheet with parchment paper. Trim the woody ends off asparagus spears and arrange them in a single layer on the prepared baking sheet. Toss cherry tomatoes with olive oil, balsamic vinegar, minced garlic, salt, and pepper until well coated, then scatter them around the asparagus on the baking sheet. Roast in the preheated oven for 15-20 minutes, or until the asparagus is tender and the tomatoes are blistered. Serve hot as a delicious and colorful side dish that's sure to impress.

Flavorful Cauliflower Creations

Cauliflower is a versatile vegetable that can be transformed into a variety of delicious low-carb side dishes. From cauliflower rice pilaf to cheesy cauliflower mash and buffalo cauliflower bites, there's a cauliflower creation to suit every taste preference.

Cauliflower Rice Pilaf with Mixed Herbs

Cauliflower rice pilaf with mixed herbs is a light and flavorful side dish that pairs well with a variety of main courses. To make this dish, start by pulsing cauliflower florets in a food processor until they resemble rice grains. Heat olive oil in a skillet over medium heat and sauté minced garlic until fragrant. Add the cauliflower rice to the skillet and cook until tender, stirring occasionally. Stir in chopped mixed herbs (such as parsley, chives, and dill) and season with salt and pepper to taste. Serve hot as a delicious and nutritious alternative to traditional rice pilaf.

Cheesy Cauliflower Mash

Cheesy cauliflower mash is a creamy and indulgent side dish that's perfect for low-carb meals. To make this dish, start by steaming or boiling cauliflower florets until tender. Drain the cauliflower and transfer it to a food processor or blender. Add butter, heavy cream, grated cheddar cheese, and minced garlic to the cauliflower, then blend until smooth and creamy. Season with salt and pepper to taste, then serve hot as a delicious and satisfying alternative to mashed potatoes.

Buffalo Cauliflower Bites with Ranch Dip

Buffalo cauliflower bites with ranch dip are a flavorful and satisfying side dish or appetizer that's perfect for game day or any gathering. To make this dish, start by preheating your oven to 450°F (230°C) and lining a baking sheet with parchment paper. Cut cauliflower into florets and toss them with olive oil, garlic powder, and salt until well coated. Spread the cauliflower out in an even layer on the prepared baking sheet and roast in the preheated oven for 20-25 minutes, or until golden brown and crispy. Meanwhile, prepare the buffalo sauce by combining melted butter and hot sauce in a bowl. Toss the roasted cauliflower with the buffalo sauce until well coated, then serve hot with ranch dip for dipping.

Fresh and Vibrant Salads

Salads are a refreshing and nutritious side dish that can be customized with a variety of ingredients to suit your taste preferences. From cucumber tomato salad with feta and olives to spinach salad with bacon and avocado, there's a salad option to complement any meal.

Cucumber Tomato Salad with Feta and Olives

Cucumber tomato salad with feta and olives is a fresh and vibrant side dish that's perfect for summer meals. To make this salad, start by thinly slicing cucumber and cherry tomatoes and placing them in a large bowl. Add sliced red onion, crumbled feta cheese, pitted Kalamata olives, and chopped fresh parsley to the bowl. Drizzle with olive oil and red wine vinegar, then season with salt and pepper to taste. Toss everything together until well combined, then serve chilled as a delicious and refreshing side dish.

Spinach Salad with Bacon and Avocado

Spinach salad with bacon and avocado is a hearty and satisfying side dish that's perfect for any occasion. To make this salad, start by cooking bacon until crispy, then crumble it into bite-sized pieces. Place baby spinach leaves in a large bowl and top with sliced avocado, cherry tomatoes, thinly sliced red onion, and the crumbled bacon. Drizzle with balsamic vinaigrette or your favorite dressing, then toss everything together until well coated. Serve immediately as a delicious and nutritious side dish that's sure to please.

Caprese Salad with Balsamic Glaze

Caprese salad with balsamic glaze is a classic Italian dish that's simple yet delicious. To make this salad, start by slicing fresh tomatoes and fresh mozzarella cheese into thick slices. Arrange the tomato and mozzarella slices on a serving platter, alternating them and overlapping slightly. Top each slice with a fresh basil leaf, then drizzle with balsamic glaze and extra virgin olive oil. Season with salt and pepper to taste, then serve immediately as a light and refreshing side dish that's perfect for any meal.

In conclusion, these tasty low-carb side dishes are perfect for adding flavor, texture, and nutrition to your meals. Whether you prefer simple roasted vegetables, flavorful cauliflower creations, or fresh and vibrant salads, there's a side dish option to suit every taste preference and dietary need.

CHAPTER SIX

Delicious Low-Carb Desserts

Indulging in desserts while sticking to a low-carb lifestyle is entirely possible with the right recipes. From decadent chocolate treats to fruity delights without the sugar and creamy dreamy desserts, there's a wide array of delicious options to satisfy your sweet tooth guilt-free.

Decadent Chocolate Treats

Who can resist the allure of rich, decadent chocolate desserts? These low-carb options will satisfy your chocolate cravings without derailing your diet.

Keto Chocolate Avocado Mousse

Keto chocolate avocado mousse is a creamy and indulgent dessert that's perfect for satisfying your chocolate cravings while staying on track with your low-carb goals. To make this mousse, start by blending ripe avocados, unsweetened cocoa powder, a low-carb sweetener of your choice (such as erythritol or stevia), vanilla extract, and a pinch of salt in a food processor or blender until smooth and creamy. Taste and adjust the sweetness as needed. Divide the mousse into individual serving cups and chill in the refrigerator for at least an hour to firm up. Serve cold with a dollop of whipped cream or coconut whipped cream for an extra indulgent treat.

Chocolate peanut butter fat bombs are a satisfying and delicious snack or dessert that's perfect for anyone following a low-carb or ketogenic diet. To make these fat bombs, start by melting unsweetened chocolate and coconut oil together in a double boiler or microwave. Stir in natural peanut butter and a low-carb sweetener of your choice (such as powdered erythritol or stevia) until smooth and well combined. Pour the mixture into silicone molds or mini muffin tins, then freeze until firm. Once set, remove the fat bombs from the molds and store them in an airtight container in the freezer until ready to enjoy. These chocolate peanut butter fat bombs are rich in healthy fats and protein, making them a satisfying and convenient option for curbing cravings.

Dark Chocolate Bark with Nuts and Sea Salt

Dark chocolate bark with nuts and sea salt is a simple yet sophisticated dessert that's perfect for satisfying your sweet tooth while staying on track with your low-carb goals. To make this bark, start by melting dark chocolate (at least 70% cocoa) in a double boiler or microwave. Stir in your favorite low-carb nuts and seeds (such as almonds, walnuts, pecans, or pumpkin seeds) until well coated. Spread the mixture out in an even layer on a parchment-lined baking sheet, then sprinkle with flaky sea salt. Chill in the refrigerator until set, then break into pieces and serve.

This dark chocolate bark is rich in antioxidants and heart-healthy fats, making it a delicious and nutritious option for dessert.

Fruity Delights without the Sugar

If you're craving something fruity but want to avoid added sugars, these low-carb desserts are perfect for you.

Mixed Berry Chia Seed Pudding

Mixed berry chia seed pudding is a refreshing and nutritious dessert that's perfect for anyone following a low-carb or ketogenic diet. To make this pudding, start by blending mixed berries (such as strawberries, blueberries, and raspberries) with unsweetened almond milk or coconut milk until smooth. Stir in chia seeds and a low-carb sweetener of your choice (such as liquid stevia or powdered erythritol) until well combined. Divide the mixture into individual serving cups or jars and chill in the refrigerator for at least two hours, or until thickened. Serve cold with fresh berries and a sprinkle of shredded coconut or chopped nuts for added texture and flavor. This mixed berry chia seed pudding is rich in fiber, antioxidants, and healthy fats, making it a delicious and satisfying dessert option.

Sugar-Free Raspberry Cheesecake Bites

Sugar-free raspberry cheesecake bites are a decadent and indulgent dessert that's perfect for satisfying your sweet tooth without derailing your low-carb lifestyle. To make these cheesecake bites, start by blending cream cheese, Greek yogurt, a low-carb sweetener of your choice (such as powdered erythritol or stevia), and vanilla extract in a food processor or blender until smooth and creamy. Divide the mixture into individual silicone molds or mini muffin tins, then top each with a fresh raspberry. Chill in the refrigerator for at least two hours, or until set. Once set, remove the cheesecake bites from the molds and serve chilled. These sugar-free raspberry cheesecake bites are rich in protein and calcium, making them a satisfying and nutritious dessert option.

Keto Lemon Bars with Almond Flour Crust

Keto lemon bars with almond flour crust are a tangy and refreshing dessert that's perfect for anyone following a low-carb or ketogenic diet. To make these bars, start by mixing almond flour, melted butter, a low-carb sweetener of your choice (such as powdered erythritol or stevia), and a pinch of salt until well combined. Press the mixture into the bottom of a parchment-lined baking dish, then bake in a preheated oven until golden brown. Meanwhile, prepare the lemon filling by whisking together eggs, lemon juice, lemon zest, a low-carb sweetener, and almond flour until smooth. Pour the filling over the baked crust and return to the oven to bake until set. Once cooled, slice into bars and dust with powdered erythritol for garnish. These keto lemon bars are bursting with citrus flavor and are sure to satisfy your dessert cravings without the guilt.

Creamy and Dreamy Desserts

Indulge in these creamy and dreamy desserts without worrying about the carb count.

Coconut Milk Panna Cotta with Berries

Coconut milk panna cotta with berries is a creamy and indulgent dessert that's perfect for anyone following a low-carb or dairy-free diet. To make this panna cotta, start by blooming gelatin in cold water until softened. Meanwhile, heat coconut milk, a low-carb sweetener of your choice (such as powdered erythritol or stevia), and vanilla extract in a saucepan until steaming but not boiling. Remove from heat and stir in the softened gelatin until dissolved. Divide the mixture into individual serving cups or ramekins and chill in the refrigerator for at least four hours, or until set. Serve cold with fresh berries and a drizzle of sugar-free berry sauce for a delicious and elegant dessert.

Vanilla Greek Yogurt with Almond Butter Drizzle

Vanilla Greek yogurt with almond butter drizzle is a creamy and satisfying dessert that's perfect for anyone following a low-carb or high-protein diet. To make this dessert, start by mixing Greek yogurt, vanilla extract, and a low-carb sweetener of your choice (such as powdered erythritol or stevia) until well combined. Divide the yogurt into individual serving cups or bowls, then drizzle with melted almond butter. Serve immediately as a delicious and nutritious dessert that's rich in protein and healthy fats.

Keto Tiramisu with Mascarpone and Espresso

Keto tiramisu with mascarpone and espresso is a rich and indulgent dessert that's perfect for special occasions or when you're craving something decadent. To make this tiramisu, start by brewing strong espresso and allowing it to cool to room temperature. Meanwhile, whip heavy cream until stiff peaks form, then fold in mascarpone cheese, a low-carb sweetener of your choice (such as powdered erythritol or stevia), and vanilla extract until smooth and creamy. Dip low-carb ladyfinger cookies (such as almond flour or coconut flour cookies) into the cooled espresso and layer them in the bottom of a serving dish. Spread a layer of the mascarpone mixture over the cookies, then repeat the layers until you reach the top of the dish. Dust the top with cocoa powder for garnish, then chill in the refrigerator for at least four hours, or until set. Serve cold as a luxurious and indulgent dessert that's sure to impress.

In conclusion, these delicious low-carb desserts prove that you can indulge your sweet tooth without derailing your diet. Whether you're craving decadent chocolate treats, fruity delights without the sugar, or creamy dreamy desserts, there's a low-carb option to satisfy every craving.

CHAPTER SEVEN

Low-Carb Snacks for Anytime

When hunger strikes between meals, having low-carb snacks on hand can help keep you satisfied and on track with your dietary goals. Whether you're looking for something crunchy, fresh, or protein-packed, these snack ideas are perfect for satisfying your cravings anytime, anywhere.

Crunchy Nut and Seed Mixes

Crunchy nut and seed mixes are perfect for satisfying your snack cravings while providing a satisfying crunch and a dose of healthy fats.

Spicy Keto Trail Mix with Nuts and Seeds

Spicy keto trail mix with nuts and seeds is a flavorful and satisfying snack that's perfect for on-the-go. To make this trail mix, combine a variety of nuts and seeds such as almonds, walnuts, pecans, pumpkin seeds, and sunflower seeds in a bowl. Toss with olive oil, smoked paprika, garlic powder, cayenne pepper, and salt until well coated. Spread the mixture out in an even layer on a baking sheet and roast in the oven at 325°F (160°C) for 15-20 minutes, stirring halfway through, until golden brown and fragrant. Let cool completely before transferring to an airtight container for storage. Pack a handful of this spicy keto trail mix for a flavorful and satisfying snack anytime you need a pick-me-up.

Almond Butter Energy Balls with Coconut

Almond butter energy balls with coconut are a nutritious and delicious snack that's perfect for satisfying your sweet tooth while providing a boost of energy. To make these energy balls, combine almond butter, unsweetened shredded coconut, ground flaxseed, chia seeds, a low-carb sweetener of your choice (such as powdered erythritol or stevia), and a splash of vanilla extract in a bowl. Stir until well combined, then roll the mixture into bite-sized balls. Roll the balls in additional shredded coconut for coating, then chill in the refrigerator for at least 30 minutes to firm up. Store the energy balls in an airtight container in the refrigerator for up to a week, or freeze for longer storage. Enjoy these almond butter energy balls as a convenient and satisfying snack anytime you need a quick pick-me-up.

Crunchy Roasted Chickpeas with Sea Salt

Crunchy roasted chickpeas with sea salt are a flavorful and satisfying snack that's perfect for munching on anytime you need a crunchy fix. To make these roasted chickpeas, start by draining and rinsing canned chickpeas and patting them dry with paper towels. Toss the chickpeas with olive oil, sea salt, and your favorite spices (such as garlic powder, cumin, or paprika) until well coated. Spread the chickpeas out in an even layer on a baking sheet and roast in the oven at 400°F (200°C) for 20-25 minutes, shaking the pan occasionally, until crispy and golden brown. Let cool completely before transferring to an airtight container for storage. Enjoy these crunchy roasted chickpeas as a delicious and nutritious snack anytime you're craving something crunchy.

Fresh and Satisfying Veggie Snacks

Fresh and satisfying veggie snacks are perfect for when you're craving something light and refreshing.

Celery Sticks with Cream Cheese and Everything Bagel Seasoning

Celery sticks with cream cheese and everything bagel seasoning are a crunchy and flavorful snack that's perfect for satisfying your cravings anytime you need a quick pick-me-up. To make these snack, spread cream cheese on celery sticks and sprinkle with everything bagel seasoning for a delicious and satisfying snack that's perfect for munching on anytime you need a quick boost of energy.

Cucumber Slices with Guacamole

Cucumber slices with guacamole are a refreshing and nutritious snack that's perfect for satisfying your cravings while providing a dose of healthy fats and fiber. To make this snack, slice cucumbers into rounds and top each with a dollop of guacamole for a delicious and satisfying snack that's perfect for munching on anytime you need a quick pick-me-up.

Bell Pepper Strips with Hummus

Bell pepper strips with hummus are a crunchy and flavorful snack that's perfect for satisfying your cravings while providing a dose of vitamins and minerals. To make this snack, slice bell peppers into strips and serve with hummus for a delicious and satisfying snack that's perfect for munching on anytime you need a quick pick-me-up.

Protein-Packed Snack Ideas

Protein-packed snack ideas are perfect for satisfying your hunger and keeping you fueled throughout the day.

Hard-Boiled Eggs with Everything Bagel Seasoning

Hard-boiled eggs with everything bagel seasoning are a nutritious and satisfying snack that's perfect for satisfying your cravings while providing a dose of protein and essential nutrients. To make this snack, hard-boil eggs and sprinkle with everything bagel seasoning for a delicious and satisfying snack that's perfect for munching on anytime you need a quick pick-me-up.

Turkey and Cheese Roll-Ups with Mustard

Turkey and cheese roll-ups with mustard are a delicious and satisfying snack that's perfect for satisfying your cravings while providing a dose of protein and calcium. To make this snack, roll slices of turkey and cheese together and serve with mustard for a delicious and satisfying snack that's perfect for munching on anytime you need a quick pick-me-up.

Greek Yogurt with Berries and a Sprinkle of Cinnamon

Greek yogurt with berries and a sprinkle of cinnamon is a creamy and delicious snack that's perfect for satisfying your cravings while providing a dose of protein and antioxidants. To make this snack, top Greek yogurt with fresh berries and a sprinkle of cinnamon for a delicious and satisfying snack that's perfect for munching on anytime you need a quick pick-me-up.

In conclusion, these low-carb snacks are perfect for satisfying your cravings anytime you need a quick pick-me-up. Whether you're craving something crunchy, fresh, or protein-packed, these snack ideas are sure to keep you satisfied and on track with your low-carb lifestyle.

CHAPTER EIGHT

Low-Carb Dining Out and Socializing

Maintaining a low-carb lifestyle doesn't have to mean missing out on social events or dining out with friends and family. With some strategic planning and mindful choices, you can enjoy socializing while staying true to your health goals.

Making Healthy Choices at Restaurants

When dining out, making healthy choices is essential to staying on track with your low-carb diet.

Opting for Grilled Proteins and Non-Starchy Vegetables

When perusing the menu, look for options that feature grilled proteins like chicken, fish, or steak, paired with non-starchy vegetables such as broccoli, asparagus, or salad greens. These choices are typically lower in carbohydrates and higher in protein and fiber, helping to keep you full and satisfied without derailing your diet.

Requesting Sauces and Dressings on the Side

Many restaurant dishes come smothered in sauces or dressings that can be high in hidden sugars and carbs. To control your intake, request sauces and dressings on the side, allowing you to add them sparingly or omit them altogether. This simple adjustment can significantly reduce the carb content of your meal while still allowing you to enjoy the flavors.

Substituting Side Dishes for Salad or Extra Vegetables

Instead of defaulting to carb-heavy side dishes like rice, potatoes, or bread, ask if you can substitute them for a side salad or extra vegetables. Most restaurants are happy to accommodate such requests, and you'll end up with a more balanced and lower-carb meal.

Navigating Social Gatherings with Ease

Social gatherings can present challenges for those following a low-carb diet, but with a bit of planning, you can navigate them with ease.

Bringing a Low-Carb Dish to Share

If you're attending a potluck or gathering where food will be served, consider bringing a low-carb dish to share. This ensures that you'll have at least one option that aligns with your dietary preferences, and it's an opportunity to introduce others to delicious low-carb recipes.

Moderating Alcohol Consumption

Alcoholic beverages can be sneaky sources of carbs, so it's essential to moderate your consumption when socializing. Opt for dry wines, spirits, or low-carb beer options, and avoid sugary mixers or cocktails. Remember to stay hydrated by alternating alcoholic drinks with water to help prevent dehydration and mitigate the effects of alcohol on your blood sugar levels.

Explaining Dietary Needs to Hosts or Friends

If you're attending a gathering hosted by friends or family, don't hesitate to communicate your dietary needs politely. Most hosts are understanding and accommodating, and they'll appreciate knowing in advance so they can plan accordingly. Offer to bring a dish to share or provide suggestions for low-carb options that you can enjoy.

Enjoying Special Occasions without Sacrificing Health Goals

Special occasions like parties or events are meant to be enjoyed, and you can still partake in the festivities while prioritizing your health goals.

Choosing Low-Carb Options at Parties and Events

Scan the buffet or appetizer spread for low-carb options like vegetable crudités with dip, cheese platters, or protein-based dishes. Fill your plate with these choices first to help curb hunger and reduce the temptation to indulge in higher-carb offerings.

Sipping on Low-Carb Cocktails or Mocktails

If cocktails are part of the celebration, opt for low-carb options like vodka soda with a splash of lime, gin and tonic with sugar-free tonic water, or a glass of dry wine. Alternatively, enjoy a refreshing mocktail made with sparkling water, fresh herbs, and citrus for a flavorful and hydrating beverage.

Focusing on Socializing and Enjoying Company Rather Than Food

Ultimately, the purpose of social gatherings is to connect with others and enjoy each other's company. Shift your focus away from the food and toward meaningful conversations, engaging activities, or simply being present in the moment. By prioritizing socializing over food, you can fully enjoy the experience without sacrificing your health goals.

In conclusion, navigating dining out and socializing while following a low-carb diet is entirely manageable with some strategic planning and mindful choices. Whether you're dining at a restaurant, attending a social gathering, or celebrating a special occasion, there are plenty of ways to enjoy yourself while staying true to your dietary preferences and health goals.

CHAPTER NINE

Planning and Preparing Low-Carb Meals

Successfully adhering to a low-carb diet often hinges on effective planning and preparation. By strategically mapping out your meals, shopping wisely, and utilizing time-saving techniques, you can make low-carb cooking a seamless and enjoyable part of your routine.

Creating Weekly Meal Plans

Developing a weekly meal plan sets the foundation for a successful low-carb diet by ensuring you have nutritious and satisfying meals ready to go.

Mapping Out Breakfast, Lunch, Dinner, and Snacks

Start by outlining each meal and snack for the week, considering your dietary preferences, nutritional needs, and schedule. Aim for a balance of protein, healthy fats, and non-starchy vegetables to keep you energized and satisfied throughout the day.

Preparing a Shopping List Based on Meal Plans

Once your meal plan is in place, compile a comprehensive shopping list of all the ingredients you'll need for the week. Organize the list by food categories to streamline your shopping trip and minimize the chances of forgetting essential items.

Batch Cooking and Meal Prepping for Busy Days

Spend some time batch cooking and meal prepping on the weekends to set yourself up for success during busy weekdays. Prepare large batches of protein, vegetables, and grains (if allowed on your low-carb plan) that can be portioned out and stored for easy reheating and assembly throughout the week.

Budget-Friendly Low-Carb Cooking

Eating low-carb doesn't have to break the bank. With strategic planning and shopping, you can enjoy nutritious meals while staying within your budget.

Choosing Inexpensive Ingredients like Frozen Vegetables or Canned Fish

Opt for budget-friendly ingredients such as frozen vegetables, canned fish (like tuna or salmon), and eggs, which offer excellent nutritional value at a fraction of the cost of fresh produce or meat. These pantry staples are versatile and can be incorporated into a wide variety of low-carb dishes.

Utilizing Leftovers in Creative Ways

Maximize your food budget by repurposing leftovers into new meals. For example, roast a whole chicken for dinner one night, then use the leftover meat to make chicken salad for lunches or shred it to top salads or soups throughout the week.

Planning Meals Around Sales and Discounts

Keep an eye on sales and discounts at your local grocery store and plan your meals accordingly. Stock up on items that are on sale or in-season produce to save money while still enjoying fresh and flavorful ingredients.

Time-Saving Tips for Effortless Low-Carb Meals

Incorporating time-saving strategies into your meal prep routine can make low-carb cooking more efficient and manageable, even on busy days.

Utilizing Kitchen Gadgets like Slow Cookers or Instant Pots

Invest in kitchen gadgets like slow cookers or Instant Pots to streamline meal preparation. These appliances allow you to set and forget your meals, saving you time and effort while still yielding delicious and nutritious results.

Streamlining Recipes with Minimal Ingredients and Prep Time

Choose recipes that require minimal ingredients and prep time to simplify your cooking process. Look for one-pot meals, sheet pan dinners, or stir-fries that can be quickly assembled and cooked with minimal fuss.

Prepping Ingredients in Advance for Quick Assembly

Prep ingredients in advance to speed up meal assembly during the week. Wash, chop, and portion out vegetables, marinate proteins, and pre-measure ingredients so they're ready to go when you need them.

By implementing these planning and preparation strategies, you can make low-carb cooking a seamless and sustainable part of your lifestyle. With careful consideration of your nutritional needs, budget, and time constraints, you can enjoy delicious and nutritious meals that support your health and wellness goals.

CHAPTER TEN

Long-Term Success with Low-Carb Diabetic Lifestyle

Achieving long-term success with a low-carb diabetic lifestyle involves more than just dietary changes. It requires setting realistic goals, building support systems, and finding balance and enjoyment in the journey towards better health.

Setting Realistic Goals and Tracking Progress

Establishing achievable health goals and tracking your progress is crucial for staying motivated and focused on your journey.

Establishing Achievable Health Goals

Set specific, measurable, and realistic health goals that align with your low-carb diabetic lifestyle. Whether it's achieving target blood sugar levels, losing weight, or improving overall well-being, having clear objectives will help guide your actions and keep you on track.

Using Apps or Journals to Monitor Food Intake and Blood Sugar

Utilize technology or traditional methods like food journals to track your food intake, blood sugar levels, and progress towards your goals. There are many apps available that can help you log meals, monitor blood glucose, and analyze nutritional data, providing valuable insights into your dietary habits and health outcomes.

Celebrating Milestones and Progress

Celebrate milestones and progress along the way to acknowledge your hard work and dedication. Whether it's reaching a weight loss milestone, achieving stable blood sugar levels, or mastering a new low-carb recipe, take the time to recognize and reward your achievements.

Building Support and Accountability

Having a strong support system and accountability partners can make a significant difference in your long-term success with a low-carb diabetic lifestyle.

Sharing Goals with Family or Friends for Support

Communicate your health goals with your family and friends to enlist their support and encouragement. Having loved ones on board can provide invaluable emotional support and motivation to stick to your low-carb plan, especially during challenging times.

Joining Online Communities or Support Groups for Encouragement

Seek out online communities or support groups comprised of individuals with similar health goals and experiences. These communities can offer a sense of belonging, empathy, and practical advice, providing a source of encouragement and motivation on your journey.

Seeking Professional Guidance from Healthcare Providers or Dietitians

Consult with healthcare providers or dietitians who specialize in diabetes management to receive personalized guidance and support. They can offer expert advice on meal planning, blood sugar management, medication adjustments, and lifestyle modifications tailored to your specific needs and preferences.

Maintaining Balance and Enjoyment in the Journey

Maintaining balance and enjoyment in your low-carb diabetic lifestyle is essential for long-term sustainability and overall well-being.

Embracing Flexibility in Eating Patterns

Practice flexibility in your eating patterns, allowing for occasional indulgences and adjustments as needed. Strive for consistency in making healthy choices most of the time while recognizing that perfection is not necessary for progress.

Incorporating Physical Activity for Overall Well-Being

Incorporate regular physical activity into your routine to support overall health and well-being. Aim for a combination of aerobic exercise, strength training, and flexibility exercises to improve insulin sensitivity, manage weight, and reduce the risk of complications associated with diabetes.

Finding Joy in Cooking and Experimenting with Low-Carb Recipes

Rediscover the joy of cooking and experimenting with low-carb recipes that are delicious, satisfying, and nourishing. Explore new ingredients, cuisines, and cooking techniques to keep meals exciting and enjoyable, making healthy eating a sustainable and fulfilling part of your lifestyle.

By setting realistic goals, building a supportive network, and maintaining balance and enjoyment in your journey, you can achieve long-term success with a low-carb diabetic lifestyle. Remember to celebrate your progress, seek professional guidance when needed, and embrace the journey towards better health and well-being.

CHAPTER 11

DIET FOR DIABETES

Pescatarian Diet:

Definition:

The pescatarian diet is a plant-based eating pattern that includes fish and seafood but excludes other animal meats such as poultry, beef, and pork. It's a flexible approach to eating that emphasizes plant foods such as fruits, vegetables, whole grains, legumes, nuts, and seeds, while also incorporating fish and seafood for protein and essential nutrients like omega-3 fatty acids.

Ingredients:

- Fish and Seafood: Salmon, trout, tuna, mackerel, shrimp, scallops, etc.

- Plant-Based Foods: Fruits, vegetables, whole grains, legumes, nuts, seeds.

- Dairy and Eggs: Milk, cheese, yogurt, eggs (optional, depending on individual preferences).

- Healthy Fats: Avocado, olive oil, nuts, seeds.

- Herbs and Spices: Basil, oregano, garlic, turmeric, ginger, etc.

Instructions/How to Prepare:

1. Base meals around plant-based foods such as fruits, vegetables, whole grains, legumes, nuts, and seeds.

2. Incorporate fish and seafood into meals as the primary source of protein.

3. Choose fatty fish like salmon, mackerel, and trout for their omega-3 fatty acids.

4. Include dairy products and eggs if desired and tolerated, as they provide additional protein and nutrients.

5. Use healthy fats like avocado, olive oil, nuts, and seeds for cooking and dressing.

6. Experiment with a variety of cooking methods, such as grilling, baking, steaming, and sautéing, to enhance flavor and texture.

7. Be mindful of portion sizes and aim for balanced meals that include a variety of food groups.

8. Opt for whole, minimally processed foods and limit intake of processed and refined foods.

9. Stay hydrated by drinking plenty of water throughout the day.

10. Consider supplementing with vitamin B12 and vitamin D if fish and seafood are the primary sources of these nutrients in the diet.

Nordic Diet:

Definition:

The Nordic diet is a traditional eating pattern inspired by the cuisines of countries in the Nordic region, such as Denmark, Finland, Iceland, Norway, and Sweden. It emphasizes seasonal, locally sourced foods that are typical of the region, including fish, seafood, whole grains, berries, root vegetables, legumes, and rapeseed oil. The diet is characterized by its high fiber, low glycemic index, and focus on quality ingredients.

Ingredients:

- Fish and Seafood: Salmon, herring, mackerel, cod, trout, shrimp, etc.

- Whole Grains: Rye bread, barley, oats, quinoa, whole grain pasta.

- Berries: Blueberries, lingonberries, raspberries, cloudberries, etc.

- Vegetables: Root vegetables (e.g., carrots, potatoes, beets), leafy greens, cabbage, onions, etc.

- Legumes: Beans, lentils, peas.

- Rapeseed Oil: Used for cooking and dressing.

- Dairy: Milk, cheese, yogurt (in moderation).

- Herbs and Spices: Dill, parsley, thyme, juniper berries, etc.

Instructions/How to Prepare:

1. Base meals around seasonal, locally sourced foods typical of the Nordic region.

2. Include fish and seafood as the primary sources of protein, aiming for 2-3 servings per week.

3. Incorporate whole grains such as rye bread, barley, oats, and quinoa into meals for fiber and nutrients.

4. Enjoy a variety of berries, which are rich in antioxidants and vitamins.

5. Include plenty of vegetables, particularly root vegetables, leafy greens, and cabbage.

6. Incorporate legumes like beans, lentils, and peas into soups, stews, and salads for plant-based protein and fiber.

7. Use rapeseed oil for cooking and dressing, as it's a traditional oil in Nordic cuisine and rich in omega-3 fatty acids.

8. Include dairy products like milk, cheese, and yogurt in moderation, opting for low-fat or fermented varieties.

9. Flavor dishes with traditional Nordic herbs and spices like dill, parsley, thyme, and juniper berries.

10.   Be mindful of portion sizes and aim for balanced meals that include a variety of food groups, focusing on quality ingredients and seasonal produce.

Asian Diet:

Definition:

The Asian diet refers to the traditional eating patterns of countries in the Asian continent, which vary greatly depending on the region and cultural influences. However, some common characteristics include a high consumption of plant-based foods such as fruits, vegetables, whole grains, legumes, and nuts; moderate intake of lean proteins such as fish, poultry, tofu, and eggs; and limited consumption of red meat and processed foods. The Asian diet is known for its emphasis on balance, variety, and moderation, as well as the inclusion of herbs, spices, and fermented foods for flavor and health benefits.

Ingredients:

- Rice: White rice, brown rice, jasmine rice, basmati rice, etc.
- Vegetables: Leafy greens, bok choy, broccoli, cabbage, carrots, onions, garlic, etc.
- Seafood: Fish, shrimp, crab, squid, mussels, etc.
- Poultry: Chicken, duck, turkey (in moderation).

- Tofu and Soy Products: Tofu, tempeh, edamame, soy milk, etc.

- Fruits: Mangoes, papayas, lychees, durian, bananas, etc.

- Nuts and Seeds: Peanuts, cashews, almonds, sesame seeds, etc.

- Herbs and Spices: Ginger, garlic, turmeric, coriander, cumin, chili peppers, etc.

- Fermented Foods: Kimchi, miso, soy sauce, fermented tofu, pickled vegetables, etc.

Instructions/How to Prepare:

1. Base meals around rice, noodles, or other staple grains, which serve as the foundation of many Asian dishes.

2. Include a variety of colorful vegetables in meals for added vitamins, minerals, and fiber.

3. Incorporate seafood, poultry, tofu, or soy products as sources of protein, aiming for a balance between plant-based and animal-based proteins.

4. Use herbs, spices, and aromatics like ginger, garlic, turmeric, and chili peppers to add flavor to dishes without relying on added fats or sodium.

5. Opt for cooking methods such as stir-frying, steaming, boiling, and grilling to retain nutrients and minimize added fats.

6. Include fermented foods like kimchi, miso, and soy sauce for their probiotic and digestive health benefits.

7. Enjoy fruits and nuts as snacks or dessert options, incorporating them into meals for added sweetness and crunch.

8. Be mindful of portion sizes and avoid overeating, focusing on listening to your body's hunger and fullness cues.

9. Stay hydrated by drinking plenty of water, green tea, or herbal teas throughout the day.

10. Embrace the cultural diversity and culinary traditions of Asian cuisine by exploring recipes and ingredients from different regions.

Traditional Indian Diet:

Definition:

The traditional Indian diet is rooted in centuries-old culinary traditions and cultural practices, with a focus on balance, variety, and Ayurvedic principles of holistic health and wellness. It emphasizes plant-based foods such as whole grains, lentils, vegetables, fruits, nuts, and seeds, while also incorporating dairy products, lean proteins, and spices for flavor and medicinal purposes. The Indian diet is known for its use of aromatic spices, herbs, and cooking techniques that enhance both taste and nutritional value.

Ingredients:

- Whole Grains: Basmati rice, brown rice, wheat, millet, barley, quinoa, etc.

- Lentils and Legumes: Red lentils, chickpeas, black beans, mung beans, pigeon peas, etc.

- Vegetables: Spinach, potatoes, cauliflower, eggplant, okra, tomatoes, etc.

- Dairy Products: Milk, yogurt, paneer (Indian cheese), ghee (clarified butter), etc.

- Spices and Herbs: Turmeric, cumin, coriander, cardamom, cinnamon, cloves, ginger, garlic, etc.

- Fruits: Mangoes, bananas, apples, papayas, oranges, guavas, etc.

- Nuts and Seeds: Almonds, cashews, pistachios, peanuts, sesame seeds, etc.

- Lean Proteins: Chicken, fish, eggs (in moderation), tofu (less traditional), etc.

Instructions/How to Prepare:

1. Base meals around whole grains, lentils, and vegetables, which form the foundation of many traditional Indian dishes.

2. Incorporate a variety of lentils and legumes into meals for plant-based protein, fiber, and essential nutrients.

3. Use a wide array of spices and herbs to add flavor to dishes, such as turmeric, cumin, coriander, and ginger, which also offer medicinal properties.

4. Include dairy products like yogurt, paneer, and ghee for added calcium, protein, and healthy fats.

5. Opt for cooking methods such as sautéing, simmering, and pressure cooking to retain nutrients and enhance flavors.

6. Enjoy fruits as snacks or desserts, incorporating them into meals for natural sweetness and additional nutrients.

7. Include nuts and seeds in dishes or as snacks for added texture, flavor, and healthy fats.

8. Be mindful of portion sizes and avoid overeating, focusing on balanced meals that include a variety of food groups.

9. Stay hydrated by drinking water, herbal teas, or buttermilk throughout the day.

10. Embrace the cultural heritage and culinary traditions of Indian cuisine by exploring regional recipes and cooking techniques.

Low-Calorie Diet:

Definition:

A low-calorie diet is characterized by reducing daily calorie intake to create a calorie deficit, which can lead to weight loss. The focus is on consuming nutrient-dense foods that are lower in calories but still provide essential nutrients, such as vitamins, minerals, and fiber. This diet typically involves portion control, meal planning, and making healthier food choices to achieve and maintain a healthy weight.

Ingredients:

- Lean Proteins: Skinless poultry, fish, seafood, tofu, tempeh, legumes.

- Non-Starchy Vegetables: Leafy greens, broccoli, cauliflower, bell peppers, zucchini, etc.

- Whole Grains (in moderation): Quinoa, brown rice, whole wheat bread, oats, barley.

- Fruits (in moderation): Berries, apples, oranges, bananas, melons, etc.

- Healthy Fats (in moderation): Avocado, nuts, seeds, olive oil.

- Low-Calorie Flavor Enhancers: Herbs, spices, vinegar, lemon juice, mustard, hot sauce.

Instructions/How to Prepare:

1. Calculate your daily calorie needs based on your age, gender, weight, height, and activity level.

2. Set a calorie goal that creates a calorie deficit for weight loss, typically 500 to 1000 calories less than your maintenance calories.

3. Plan meals that include lean proteins, non-starchy vegetables, whole grains (in moderation), fruits (in moderation), and healthy fats (in moderation).

4. Incorporate low-calorie flavor enhancers such as herbs, spices, vinegar, lemon juice, mustard, and hot sauce to add flavor without adding extra calories.

5. Be mindful of portion sizes and avoid oversized servings, using smaller plates and utensils if necessary.

6. Focus on filling half of your plate with non-starchy vegetables to add volume and fiber to meals while keeping calories low.

7. Choose lean protein sources like skinless poultry, fish, tofu, and legumes to help satisfy hunger and maintain muscle mass.

8. Include whole grains and fruits in moderation for added nutrients and fiber, but be cautious of portion sizes to manage calorie intake.

9. Incorporate healthy fats like avocado, nuts, seeds, and olive oil into meals to promote satiety and provide essential fatty acids.

10. Stay hydrated by drinking plenty of water throughout the day, as thirst can sometimes be mistaken for hunger.

Gluten-Free Diet:

Definition:

A gluten-free diet involves eliminating foods that contain gluten, a protein found in wheat, barley, rye, and their derivatives. This diet is essential for individuals with celiac disease, an autoimmune disorder triggered by gluten, as well as those with non-celiac gluten sensitivity or wheat allergy. The gluten-free diet focuses on naturally gluten-free foods and gluten-free alternatives to grains containing gluten.

Ingredients:

- Naturally Gluten-Free Foods: Fruits, vegetables, nuts, seeds, legumes, meats, fish, seafood, eggs, dairy products.

- Gluten-Free Grains and Flours: Rice, quinoa, corn, millet, buckwheat, sorghum, amaranth, teff, gluten-free oats, almond flour, coconut flour, chickpea flour, etc.

- Gluten-Free Condiments and Flavorings: Tamari (gluten-free soy sauce), mustard, vinegar, herbs, spices, etc.

- Gluten-Free Snacks and Treats: Popcorn, rice cakes, gluten-free crackers, gluten-free cookies, dark chocolate, etc.

Instructions/How to Prepare:

1. Educate yourself about sources of gluten and read food labels carefully to identify gluten-containing ingredients.

2. Base meals around naturally gluten-free foods such as fruits, vegetables, nuts, seeds, legumes, meats, fish, seafood, eggs, and dairy products.

3. Choose gluten-free grains and flours as alternatives to wheat, barley, and rye, including rice, quinoa, corn, millet, buckwheat, and gluten-free oats.

4. Use gluten-free condiments and flavorings like tamari (gluten-free soy sauce), mustard, vinegar, herbs, and spices to add flavor to meals.

5. Be cautious of cross-contamination by using separate cooking utensils, cutting boards, and kitchen equipment for gluten-free foods.

6. Explore gluten-free alternatives to favorite dishes and snacks, such as gluten-free pasta, bread, crackers, and baked goods.

7. Experiment with gluten-free cooking and baking techniques using alternative flours like almond flour, coconut flour, and chickpea flour.

8. Be aware of hidden sources of gluten in processed foods, sauces, dressings, and packaged snacks, and choose certified gluten-free products when possible.

9. Check with restaurants about their gluten-free options and food preparation practices when dining out.

10. Consider working with a registered dietitian or healthcare professional knowledgeable about gluten-free diets to ensure nutritional adequacy and dietary compliance.

Anti-Inflammatory Diet:

Definition:

An anti-inflammatory diet focuses on reducing inflammation in the body by emphasizing foods that have been shown to have anti-inflammatory properties while limiting or avoiding those that may contribute to inflammation. Chronic inflammation is associated with various health conditions, including heart disease, diabetes, arthritis, and certain cancers. The anti-inflammatory diet typically includes a variety of whole, nutrient-rich foods such as fruits, vegetables, whole grains, healthy fats, and lean proteins, while minimizing processed foods, refined sugars, and unhealthy fats.

Ingredients:

- Fruits: Berries, cherries, oranges, pineapple, papaya, etc.

- Vegetables: Leafy greens, broccoli, Brussels sprouts, cauliflower, sweet potatoes, etc.

- Whole Grains: Quinoa, brown rice, oats, barley, bulgur, whole wheat pasta.

- Healthy Fats: Avocado, olive oil, nuts, seeds, fatty fish (salmon, mackerel, sardines).

- Lean Proteins: Skinless poultry, fish, seafood, tofu, tempeh, legumes, beans.

- Herbs and Spices: Turmeric, ginger, garlic, cinnamon, cumin, basil, oregano, etc.

Instructions/How to Prepare:

1. Base meals around whole, nutrient-rich foods such as fruits, vegetables, whole grains, healthy fats, and lean proteins.

2. Incorporate a variety of colorful fruits and vegetables into meals and snacks for their antioxidants and anti-inflammatory compounds.

3. Choose whole grains like quinoa, brown rice, and oats over refined grains for added fiber and nutrients.

4. Include healthy fats like avocado, olive oil, nuts, and seeds in moderation to reduce inflammation and support overall health.

5. Opt for lean protein sources such as fish, poultry, tofu, and legumes, which contain anti-inflammatory properties.

6. Flavor dishes with herbs and spices like turmeric, ginger, garlic, cinnamon, and cumin, which have been shown to have anti-inflammatory effects.

7. Minimize consumption of processed foods, refined sugars, and unhealthy fats, which can contribute to inflammation.

8. Be mindful of portion sizes and avoid overeating, focusing on listening to your body's hunger and fullness cues.

9. Stay hydrated by drinking plenty of water throughout the day, as dehydration can exacerbate inflammation.

10.   Aim for a balanced diet that includes a variety of nutrient-dense foods while reducing sources of inflammation, and consider consulting with a healthcare professional or registered dietitian for personalized guidance and support.

Raw Food Diet:

Definition:

The raw food diet is based on the belief that consuming foods in their natural, uncooked state provides maximum nutritional benefits and enzymes that are destroyed during cooking. This diet typically includes raw fruits, vegetables, nuts, seeds, sprouted grains, and legumes, as well as some raw or minimally processed dairy products, eggs, fish, and meat. The raw food diet is high in vitamins, minerals, fiber, and antioxidants, and proponents believe it can lead to improved digestion, increased energy, weight loss, and reduced risk of chronic diseases.

Ingredients:

- Raw Fruits: Berries, apples, oranges, bananas, mangoes, etc.

- Raw Vegetables: Leafy greens, carrots, cucumbers, bell peppers, tomatoes, etc.

- Nuts and Seeds: Almonds, walnuts, cashews, sunflower seeds, chia seeds, flaxseeds, etc.

- Sprouted Grains and Legumes: Sprouted quinoa, lentils, chickpeas, mung beans, etc.

- Raw Dairy and Eggs (if consumed): Raw milk, cheese, yogurt, eggs (in moderation).

- Raw or Minimally Processed Meat and Fish (if consumed): Sashimi, ceviche, carpaccio, etc.

- Cold-Pressed Oils: Olive oil, coconut oil, flaxseed oil, etc.

Instructions/How to Prepare:

1. Base meals around raw fruits, vegetables, nuts, seeds, sprouted grains, and legumes.

2. Incorporate a variety of colorful fruits and vegetables into meals and snacks for their vitamins, minerals, and antioxidants.

3. Include nuts and seeds for healthy fats, protein, and fiber, using them in salads, smoothies, or raw energy bars.

4. Experiment with sprouted grains and legumes, which are easier to digest and may have increased nutrient bioavailability.

5. Be cautious with raw dairy and eggs, choosing high-quality, pasteurized options to reduce the risk of foodborne illness.

6. If consuming raw meat or fish, ensure it is fresh, high-quality, and properly handled to minimize the risk of foodborne pathogens.

7. Use cold-pressed oils like olive oil, coconut oil, and flaxseed oil for dressing salads or adding flavor to dishes.

8. Be creative with food preparation techniques such as blending, juicing, dehydrating, and marinating to enhance flavor and texture.

9. Be mindful of food safety practices when handling raw foods, including washing produce thoroughly and storing perishable items properly.

10. Listen to your body and adjust the raw food diet to meet your individual nutritional needs, and consider consulting with a healthcare professional or registered dietitian for personalized guidance and support.

Specific Carbohydrate Diet (SCD):

Definition:

The Specific Carbohydrate Diet (SCD) is a dietary regimen designed to manage certain digestive disorders, particularly inflammatory bowel diseases (IBD) such as Crohn's disease, ulcerative colitis, and celiac disease. It aims to reduce inflammation and promote healing of the gastrointestinal tract by restricting certain carbohydrates that are thought to exacerbate symptoms. The diet focuses on consuming easily digestible, nutrient-rich foods that are low in carbohydrates and free of complex sugars and starches.

Ingredients:

- Fresh Fruits: Apples, bananas, berries, melons, etc.

- Non-Starchy Vegetables: Leafy greens, carrots, cucumbers, bell peppers, squash, etc.

- Lean Proteins: Chicken, turkey, fish, eggs, tofu, tempeh, and certain cuts of beef or pork.

- Healthy Fats: Olive oil, coconut oil, avocados, nuts, seeds.

- Fermented Foods (in moderation): Yogurt, kefir, sauerkraut, kimchi.

- Certain Legumes and Beans (in limited amounts): Lentils, black beans, navy beans.

- Homemade Broths and Soups: Chicken broth, bone broth, vegetable soup.

- Natural Sweeteners (in moderation): Honey, maple syrup.

Instructions/How to Prepare:

1. Eliminate complex carbohydrates such as grains, processed foods, and sugars from the diet.

2. Base meals around fresh fruits, non-starchy vegetables, lean proteins, and healthy fats.

3. Choose easily digestible proteins such as poultry, fish, eggs, tofu, and tempeh.

4. Incorporate healthy fats like olive oil, coconut oil, avocados, nuts, and seeds into meals for satiety and energy.

5. Include fermented foods like yogurt, kefir, sauerkraut, and kimchi in moderation to support gut health and digestion.

6. Experiment with homemade broths and soups made from scratch using nutrient-rich ingredients.

7. Be cautious with certain legumes and beans, as they may cause digestive discomfort in some individuals.

8. Use natural sweeteners like honey and maple syrup sparingly, as they are allowed in moderation on the SCD.

9. Avoid processed foods, artificial additives, and preservatives, opting for whole, unprocessed foods whenever possible.

10. Monitor symptoms and adjust the diet as needed to manage digestive issues and promote overall well-being, and consider consulting with a healthcare professional or registered dietitian for personalized guidance and support.

Zone Diet:

Definition:

The Zone Diet is a low-glycemic, moderate-protein, and moderate-fat eating plan designed to optimize hormone levels, promote weight loss, and improve overall health and performance. It aims to balance macronutrients in a specific ratio to control inflammation, stabilize blood sugar levels, and enhance metabolic function. The diet emphasizes portion control and consuming meals that are rich in protein, low in carbohydrates, and include healthy fats to maintain a state of "the zone," where the body efficiently burns fat for fuel.

Ingredients:

- Lean Proteins: Skinless poultry, fish, seafood, tofu, tempeh, lean cuts of beef or pork.

- Non-Starchy Vegetables: Leafy greens, broccoli, cauliflower, bell peppers, zucchini, spinach, etc.

- Healthy Fats: Olive oil, avocado, nuts, seeds, fatty fish (salmon, mackerel, sardines).

- Low-Glycemic Carbohydrates (in moderation): Berries, apples, oranges, quinoa, brown rice, sweet potatoes.

- Some Dairy Products (in moderation): Greek yogurt, cottage cheese, low-fat cheese.

Instructions/How to Prepare:

1. Divide meals into specific portions of protein, carbohydrates, and fats to achieve the desired macronutrient ratio (40% carbohydrates, 30% protein, 30% fat).

2. Base meals around lean proteins such as poultry, fish, seafood, tofu, and tempeh, aiming for a portion size that fits in the palm of your hand.

3. Include plenty of non-starchy vegetables like leafy greens, broccoli, cauliflower, and bell peppers to bulk up meals and add fiber and nutrients.

4. Incorporate healthy fats like olive oil, avocado, nuts, and seeds into meals for satiety and to help balance blood sugar levels.

5. Choose low-glycemic carbohydrates such as berries, apples, oranges, quinoa, brown rice, and sweet potatoes to minimize spikes in blood sugar.

6. Be mindful of portion sizes and avoid overeating, focusing on balanced meals that include a variety of food groups.

7. Include some dairy products like Greek yogurt, cottage cheese, and low-fat cheese in moderation for additional protein and calcium.

8. Plan meals and snacks ahead of time to ensure they fit within the macronutrient ratio and support your nutritional goals.

9. Stay hydrated by drinking plenty of water throughout the day to support metabolic function and overall health.

10. Monitor progress and adjust portion sizes and food choices as needed to achieve and maintain the desired balance of macronutrients, and consider consulting with a healthcare professional or registered dietitian for personalized guidance and support.

Engine 2 Diet:

Definition:

The Engine 2 Diet, developed by firefighter Rip Esselstyn, is a plant-based eating plan designed to promote heart health, weight loss, and overall well-being. It emphasizes whole, nutrient-dense, plant-based foods while minimizing or eliminating animal products, oils, processed foods, and added sugars. The diet is inspired by the idea that eating "like a firefighter" – with a focus on whole plant foods – can prevent and even reverse chronic diseases such as heart disease, diabetes, and obesity.

Ingredients:

- Whole Grains: Brown rice, quinoa, oats, barley, whole wheat pasta, whole grain bread.

- Beans and Legumes: Black beans, lentils, chickpeas, kidney beans, edamame, tofu.

- Fruits: Berries, apples, oranges, bananas, mangoes, melons, etc.

- Vegetables: Leafy greens, broccoli, cauliflower, bell peppers, carrots, onions, etc.

- Nuts and Seeds (in moderation): Almonds, walnuts, chia seeds, flaxseeds, hemp seeds, etc.

- Herbs and Spices: Basil, oregano, garlic, ginger, turmeric, cumin, etc.

Instructions/How to Prepare:

1. Base meals around whole, plant-based foods such as whole grains, beans, legumes, fruits, and vegetables.

2. Include a variety of colorful fruits and vegetables in meals and snacks for their vitamins, minerals, and antioxidants.

3. Choose whole grains like brown rice, quinoa, oats, and barley for fiber and nutrients.

4. Incorporate beans and legumes into meals for plant-based protein, fiber, and essential nutrients.

5. Limit or eliminate processed foods, oils, added sugars, and animal products from the diet.

6. Use nuts and seeds sparingly for added texture and flavor, as they are high in calories.

7. Flavor dishes with herbs and spices instead of salt or added fats to enhance taste without extra calories.

8. Experiment with plant-based cooking techniques such as steaming, sautéing, roasting, and grilling to bring out natural flavors.

9. Be mindful of portion sizes and avoid overeating, focusing on balanced meals that include a variety of food groups.

10. Stay hydrated by drinking plenty of water throughout the day, and consider incorporating regular physical activity to complement dietary changes.

Dr. Bernstein's Diabetes Diet:

Definition:

Dr. Richard K. Bernstein's Diabetes Diet is a low-carbohydrate eating plan specifically designed to manage blood sugar levels and improve health outcomes for individuals with diabetes, particularly type 1 diabetes. It emphasizes controlling carbohydrate intake to prevent spikes in blood sugar, achieve stable glucose levels, and reduce the need for insulin medication. The diet consists of whole, nutrient-dense foods that are low in carbohydrates but rich in protein, healthy fats, fiber, vitamins, and minerals.

Ingredients:

- Non-Starchy Vegetables: Leafy greens, broccoli, cauliflower, bell peppers, zucchini, spinach, etc.

- Lean Proteins: Chicken, turkey, fish, seafood, eggs, tofu, tempeh, lean cuts of beef or pork.

- Healthy Fats: Olive oil, avocado, nuts, seeds, fatty fish (salmon, mackerel, sardines).

- Low-Glycemic Carbohydrates (in moderation): Berries, apples, oranges, quinoa, brown rice, sweet potatoes.

- Some Dairy Products (in moderation): Greek yogurt, cottage cheese, low-fat cheese.

Instructions/How to Prepare:

1. Limit carbohydrate intake to a specific amount per meal, typically 15 grams or less for breakfast and 30 grams or less for lunch and dinner.

2. Base meals around non-starchy vegetables, which are low in carbohydrates and high in fiber, vitamins, and minerals.

3. Include lean proteins such as poultry, fish, seafood, eggs, tofu, and tempeh in each meal to help stabilize blood sugar levels and promote satiety.

4. Incorporate healthy fats like olive oil, avocado, nuts, and seeds into meals for sustained energy and to slow the absorption of carbohydrates.

5. Choose low-glycemic carbohydrates like berries, apples, oranges, quinoa, brown rice, and sweet potatoes in moderation to minimize spikes in blood sugar.

6. Be cautious with portion sizes and avoid overeating, especially with carbohydrate-rich foods.

7. Monitor blood sugar levels regularly and adjust carbohydrate intake, insulin medication, and dietary choices as needed to maintain stable glucose levels.

8. Plan meals and snacks ahead of time to ensure they fit within the carbohydrate limits and support blood sugar control.

9. Stay hydrated by drinking plenty of water throughout the day, and consider incorporating regular physical activity to improve insulin sensitivity and overall health.

10. Work closely with a healthcare professional or registered dietitian experienced in diabetes management to develop a personalized meal plan and monitor progress over time.

Intermittent Fasting:

Definition:

Intermittent Fasting (IF) is an eating pattern that cycles between periods of fasting and eating. It doesn't prescribe specific foods to eat but rather focuses on when to eat them. There are several variations of intermittent fasting, including the 16/8 method, the 5:2 diet, alternate-day fasting, and spontaneous meal skipping. Intermittent fasting has gained popularity for its potential benefits for weight loss, improved metabolic health, and simplified eating patterns.

Instructions/How to Prepare:

1. Choose an intermittent fasting protocol that aligns with your lifestyle, preferences, and health goals.

2. In the 16/8 method, for example, you fast for 16 hours and restrict eating to an 8-hour window each day.

3. During the fasting period, consume only non-caloric beverages such as water, black coffee, or herbal tea to help control hunger and maintain hydration.

4. Plan meals and snacks to fit within the designated eating window, focusing on nutrient-dense foods to support overall health.

5. Include a variety of whole foods such as fruits, vegetables, lean proteins, healthy fats, and whole grains in meals to promote satiety and provide essential nutrients.

6. Be mindful of portion sizes and avoid overeating during the eating window to prevent excessive calorie intake.

7. Stay hydrated by drinking plenty of water throughout the fasting and eating periods to support hydration and overall well-being.

8. Listen to your body and adjust the fasting schedule as needed to accommodate changes in hunger, energy levels, and lifestyle demands.

9. Monitor progress and pay attention to how you feel physically, mentally, and emotionally while practicing intermittent fasting.

10. Consult with a healthcare professional or registered dietitian before starting intermittent fasting, especially if you have underlying health conditions or concerns about its suitability for you.

The Biggest Loser Diet:

Definition:

The Biggest Loser Diet is a weight loss program inspired by the reality TV show "The Biggest Loser," which features contestants competing to lose the most weight through diet and exercise. The diet emphasizes portion control, calorie restriction, and regular physical activity to achieve weight loss goals. It focuses on consuming lean proteins, whole grains, fruits, vegetables, and limited amounts of healthy fats while minimizing processed foods, refined sugars, and unhealthy fats.

Ingredients:

- Lean Proteins: Chicken, turkey, fish, seafood, tofu, tempeh, lean cuts of beef or pork.

- Whole Grains: Brown rice, quinoa, oats, barley, whole wheat bread, whole grain pasta.

- Fruits: Berries, apples, oranges, bananas, mangoes, melons, etc.

- Vegetables: Leafy greens, broccoli, cauliflower, bell peppers, carrots, onions, etc.

- Healthy Fats (in moderation): Avocado, nuts, seeds, olive oil.

- Low-Fat Dairy Products (in moderation): Greek yogurt, cottage cheese, skim milk.

Instructions/How to Prepare:

1. Calculate daily calorie needs based on weight loss goals, activity level, and metabolic rate.

2. Plan meals and snacks that incorporate lean proteins, whole grains, fruits, vegetables, and healthy fats within calorie limits.

3. Use portion control techniques such as measuring food portions, using smaller plates, and being mindful of serving sizes.

4. Focus on consuming nutrient-dense foods that provide essential vitamins, minerals, and antioxidants.

5. Include regular physical activity as part of the weight loss plan, incorporating a combination of cardiovascular exercise, strength training, and flexibility exercises.

6. Be mindful of fluid intake and stay hydrated by drinking plenty of water throughout the day.

7. Monitor progress by tracking food intake, exercise, and weight loss using a journal or app.

8. Practice mindful eating by paying attention to hunger and fullness cues, eating slowly, and savoring each bite.

9. Be consistent with meal planning, grocery shopping, and food preparation to support healthy eating habits.

10. Seek support from friends, family, or a weight loss group for accountability, motivation, and encouragement throughout the journey.

Weight Watchers (WW):

Definition:

Weight Watchers (WW) is a popular weight loss program that focuses on a balanced approach to eating and lifestyle changes. It assigns point values to foods based on their nutritional content, with the goal of promoting portion control, balanced nutrition, and sustainable weight loss. Participants are assigned a daily and weekly points allowance based on their age, weight, height, gender, and weight loss goals. They can choose from a wide variety of foods and are encouraged to make healthier choices, increase physical activity, and develop lifelong habits for success.

Ingredients:

- Lean Proteins: Chicken, turkey, fish, seafood, tofu, tempeh, lean cuts of beef or pork.

- Whole Grains: Brown rice, quinoa, oats, barley, whole wheat bread, whole grain pasta.

- Fruits: Berries, apples, oranges, bananas, mangoes, melons, etc.

- Vegetables: Leafy greens, broccoli, cauliflower, bell peppers, carrots, onions, etc.

- Healthy Fats: Avocado, nuts, seeds, olive oil.

- Low-Fat Dairy Products: Greek yogurt, cottage cheese, skim milk.

- Zero-Point Foods: Certain fruits, vegetables, lean proteins, and other foods with low calorie density.

Instructions/How to Prepare:

1. Join the Weight Watchers program to access personalized support, resources, and tools for weight loss success.

2. Attend group meetings, workshops, or virtual sessions for guidance, accountability, and motivation.

3. Calculate daily and weekly SmartPoints allowance based on individual factors and weight loss goals.

4. Track food intake and activity using the WW app or website, assigning point values to foods and staying within the allotted points allowance.

5. Make healthier food choices by selecting foods that are lower in points and higher in nutritional value, such as lean proteins, whole grains, fruits, and vegetables.

6. Incorporate zero-point foods into meals and snacks to increase satiety and reduce overall calorie intake.

7. Practice portion control and mindful eating by paying attention to serving sizes and eating slowly.

8. Increase physical activity by setting activity goals, incorporating regular exercise into daily routines, and finding activities that are enjoyable and sustainable.

9. Seek support from the WW community, including coaches, members, and online forums, for encouragement, advice, and inspiration.

10.   Celebrate successes, track progress, and stay committed to making healthy lifestyle changes for long-term weight management and overall well-being.

The Mayo Clinic Diet:

Definition:

The Mayo Clinic Diet is a weight loss and lifestyle program developed by the renowned Mayo Clinic. It focuses on making long-term, sustainable changes to promote healthy weight loss and improve overall health and well-being. Unlike fad diets, The Mayo Clinic Diet emphasizes practical, realistic strategies for incorporating healthy eating habits, physical activity, and positive behavior changes into daily life. The diet is divided into two phases: "Lose It!" and "Live It!" The first phase focuses on jump-starting weight loss by adopting healthy habits, while the second phase is designed to help maintain weight loss and continue making progress toward health goals.

Ingredients:

- Fruits: Berries, apples, oranges, bananas, mangoes, melons, etc.

- Vegetables: Leafy greens, broccoli, cauliflower, bell peppers, carrots, onions, etc.

- Whole Grains: Brown rice, quinoa, oats, barley, whole wheat bread, whole grain pasta.

- Lean Proteins: Chicken, turkey, fish, seafood, tofu, tempeh, lean cuts of beef or pork.

- Healthy Fats: Avocado, nuts, seeds, olive oil.

- Low-Fat Dairy Products: Greek yogurt, cottage cheese, skim milk.

Instructions/How to Prepare:

1. Set realistic weight loss and health goals based on individual preferences, needs, and medical history.

2. Adopt healthy eating habits by incorporating a variety of nutrient-rich foods such as fruits, vegetables, whole grains, lean proteins, and healthy fats into meals and snacks.

3. Focus on portion control and mindful eating by paying attention to hunger and fullness cues, eating slowly, and savoring each bite.

4. Limit or avoid processed foods, refined sugars, unhealthy fats, and excess sodium, opting for whole, minimally processed foods whenever possible.

5. Increase physical activity by setting achievable goals, incorporating regular exercise into daily routines, and finding activities that are enjoyable and sustainable.

6. Practice self-monitoring by tracking food intake, physical activity, and progress toward health goals using a journal or app.

7. Seek support from friends, family, or a weight loss group for accountability, motivation, and encouragement throughout the journey.

8. Be patient and flexible, recognizing that weight loss and lifestyle changes take time and effort, and embracing setbacks as opportunities for learning and growth.

9. Gradually transition to the "Live It!" phase of The Mayo Clinic Diet, focusing on maintaining weight loss, continuing healthy habits, and making sustainable lifestyle changes for long-term success.

10. Celebrate successes, track progress, and stay committed to making healthy choices for lifelong health and well-being.

Carbohydrate Counting Diet:

Definition:

The Carbohydrate Counting Diet is a method used by individuals with diabetes to manage blood sugar levels by closely monitoring carbohydrate intake. It involves counting the grams of carbohydrates in foods and balancing them with insulin doses or other blood sugar-lowering medications. The diet aims to provide flexibility in food choices while maintaining stable blood sugar levels throughout the day. It's commonly used by individuals with type 1 diabetes, type 2 diabetes, or gestational diabetes.

Ingredients:

- Carbohydrate-Containing Foods: Bread, rice, pasta, cereals, fruits, starchy vegetables, dairy products, legumes, sweets, and desserts.

- Non-Starchy Vegetables: Leafy greens, broccoli, cauliflower, bell peppers, zucchini, spinach, cucumber, etc.

- Lean Proteins: Chicken, turkey, fish, seafood, eggs, tofu, tempeh, lean cuts of beef or pork.

- Healthy Fats: Olive oil, avocado, nuts, seeds, fatty fish (salmon, mackerel, sardines).

- Low-Glycemic Carbohydrates (in moderation): Berries, apples, oranges, quinoa, brown rice, sweet potatoes.

- Some Dairy Products (in moderation): Greek yogurt, cottage cheese, low-fat cheese.

Instructions/How to Prepare:

1. Determine individual carbohydrate goals based on factors such as age, weight, activity level, blood sugar targets, and insulin sensitivity.

2. Learn to identify carbohydrate-containing foods and understand portion sizes to accurately count grams of carbohydrates.

3. Monitor carbohydrate intake throughout the day by reading food labels, using carbohydrate counting apps, or referring to carbohydrate counting resources.

4. Distribute carbohydrate intake evenly across meals and snacks to help stabilize blood sugar levels throughout the day.

5. Pair carbohydrates with lean proteins, healthy fats, and fiber-rich foods to slow the absorption of glucose and minimize blood sugar spikes.

6. Be mindful of high-glycemic carbohydrates and limit their intake to prevent rapid increases in blood sugar levels.

7. Consider timing carbohydrate intake around physical activity to optimize energy levels and blood sugar management.

8. Adjust insulin doses or other blood sugar-lowering medications based on carbohydrate intake and blood sugar levels, under the guidance of a healthcare professional.

9. Monitor blood sugar levels regularly and make adjustments to carbohydrate intake, insulin doses, or medication regimens as needed to maintain stable glucose levels.

10.   Work closely with a healthcare professional or registered dietitian experienced in diabetes management to develop a personalized carbohydrate counting plan and receive ongoing support and education.

CHAPTER 12

31 DAYS MEAL PLAN

Week 1:

Day 1:

- Breakfast: Scrambled eggs with spinach and mushrooms
- Lunch: Grilled chicken salad with mixed greens and vinaigrette dressing
- Dinner: Baked salmon with steamed broccoli

Day 2:

- Breakfast: Greek yogurt with berries and almonds
- Lunch: Turkey and cheese lettuce wraps with avocado
- Dinner: Cauliflower rice stir-fry with tofu and mixed vegetables

Day 3:

- Breakfast: Spinach and feta omelette
- Lunch: Tuna salad with cucumber slices
- Dinner: Grilled shrimp with zucchini noodles and marinara sauce

Day 4:

- Breakfast: Chia seed pudding with unsweetened almond milk and sliced strawberries

- Lunch: Egg salad with lettuce wraps

- Dinner: Baked chicken thighs with roasted Brussels sprouts

Day 5:

- Breakfast: Cottage cheese with sliced peaches and walnuts

- Lunch: Turkey and avocado wrap with lettuce

- Dinner: Beef stir-fry with broccoli and cauliflower rice

Day 6:

- Breakfast: Smoothie made with spinach, avocado, and unsweetened almond milk

- Lunch: Grilled chicken Caesar salad with a light dressing

- Dinner: Baked cod with asparagus

Day 7:

- Breakfast: Scrambled eggs with bell peppers and onions

- Lunch: Greek salad with grilled chicken

- Dinner: Vegetable stir-fry with tofu and cauliflower rice

Week 2:

Day 8:

- Breakfast: Greek yogurt with sliced almonds and raspberries

- Lunch: Turkey and cheese roll-ups with cucumber slices

- Dinner: Baked salmon with roasted green beans

Day 9:

- Breakfast: Spinach and cheese frittata

- Lunch: Tuna salad lettuce wraps with avocado

- Dinner: Grilled shrimp skewers with cauliflower rice

Day 10:

- Breakfast: Chia seed pudding with coconut milk and blueberries

- Lunch: Egg salad with cucumber slices

- Dinner: Baked chicken breast with sautéed spinach

Day 11:

- Breakfast: Cottage cheese with sliced strawberries and pecans

- Lunch: Turkey and avocado wrap with lettuce

- Dinner: Beef stir-fry with bell peppers and zucchini noodles

Day 12:

- Breakfast: Smoothie made with kale, berries, and unsweetened almond milk

- Lunch: Grilled chicken salad with mixed greens and vinaigrette dressing

- Dinner: Baked cod with roasted cauliflower

Day 13:

- Breakfast: Scrambled eggs with spinach and mushrooms

- Lunch: Greek salad with grilled chicken

- Dinner: Vegetable stir-fry with tofu and cauliflower rice

Day 14:

- Breakfast: Greek yogurt with sliced almonds and raspberries

- Lunch: Turkey and cheese lettuce wraps with avocado

- Dinner: Baked salmon with roasted broccoli

Week 3:

Day 15:

- Breakfast: Spinach and cheese omelette

- Lunch: Tuna salad with cucumber slices

- Dinner: Grilled shrimp with zucchini noodles and marinara sauce

Day 16:

- Breakfast: Chia seed pudding with unsweetened almond milk and sliced strawberries
- Lunch: Egg salad with lettuce wraps
- Dinner: Baked chicken thighs with roasted Brussels sprouts

Day 17:

- Breakfast: Cottage cheese with sliced peaches and walnuts
- Lunch: Turkey and avocado wrap with lettuce
- Dinner: Beef stir-fry with broccoli and cauliflower rice

Day 18:

- Breakfast: Smoothie made with spinach, avocado, and unsweetened almond milk
- Lunch: Grilled chicken Caesar salad with a light dressing
- Dinner: Baked cod with asparagus

Day 19:

- Breakfast: Scrambled eggs with bell peppers and onions
- Lunch: Greek salad with grilled chicken
- Dinner: Vegetable stir-fry with tofu and cauliflower rice

Day 20:

- Breakfast: Greek yogurt with sliced almonds and raspberries

- Lunch: Turkey and cheese roll-ups with cucumber slices

- Dinner: Baked salmon with roasted green beans

Day 21:

- Breakfast: Spinach and cheese frittata

- Lunch: Tuna salad lettuce wraps with avocado

- Dinner: Grilled shrimp skewers with cauliflower rice

Week 4:

Day 22:

- Breakfast: Chia seed pudding with coconut milk and blueberries

- Lunch: Egg salad with cucumber slices

- Dinner: Baked chicken breast with sautéed spinach

Day 23:

- Breakfast: Cottage cheese with sliced strawberries and pecans

- Lunch: Turkey and avocado wrap with lettuce

- Dinner: Beef stir-fry with bell peppers and zucchini noodles

Day 24:

- Breakfast: Smoothie made with kale, berries, and unsweetened almond milk

- Lunch: Grilled chicken salad with mixed greens and vinaigrette dressing

- Dinner: Baked cod with roasted cauliflower

Day 25:

- Breakfast: Scrambled eggs with spinach and mushrooms

- Lunch: Greek salad with grilled chicken

- Dinner: Vegetable stir-fry with tofu and cauliflower rice

Day 26:

- Breakfast: Greek yogurt with sliced almonds and raspberries

- Lunch: Turkey and cheese lettuce wraps with avocado

- Dinner: Baked salmon with roasted broccoli

Day 27:

- Breakfast: Spinach and cheese omelette

- Lunch: Tuna salad with cucumber slices

- Dinner: Grilled shrimp with zucchini noodles and marinara sauce

Day 28:

- Breakfast: Chia seed pudding with unsweetened almond milk and sliced strawberries

- Lunch: Egg salad with lettuce wraps

- Dinner: Baked chicken thighs with roasted Brussels sprouts

Day 29:

- Breakfast: Cottage cheese with sliced peaches and walnuts

- Lunch: Turkey and avocado wrap with lettuce

- Dinner: Beef stir-fry with broccoli and cauliflower rice

Day 30:

- Breakfast: Smoothie made with spinach, avocado, and unsweetened almond milk

- Lunch: Grilled chicken Caesar salad with a light dressing

- Dinner: Baked cod with asparagus

Day 31:

- Breakfast: Scrambled eggs with bell peppers and onions

- Lunch: Greek salad with grilled chicken

- Dinner: Vegetable stir-fry with tofu and cauliflower rice

THE END

www.ingramcontent.com/pod-product-compliance
Lightning Source LLC
Chambersburg PA
CBHW081550250726
48653CB00009B/3364